WITHDRAWN
UTSA LIBRARIES

RENEWALS

DE

A

A

AI

A

DI

SCHIZOPHRENIA
A Psychopharmacological Approach

Publication Number 839
AMERICAN LECTURE SERIES®

A Monograph in
AMERICAN LECTURES IN OBJECTIVE PSYCHIATRY

Edited by
WILLIAM HORSLEY GANTT, M.D.
Veterans Administration Hospital
Pavlovian Research Laboratory
Perry Point, Maryland

SCHIZOPHRENIA

A Psychopharmacological Approach

By

THOMAS A. BAN, M.D.

Director, Division of Psychopharmacology
Associate Professor of Psychiatry
McGill University
Chief, Research Services
Douglas Hospital
Montreal, Quebec, Canada

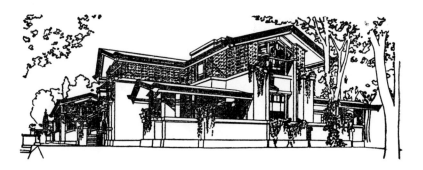

CHARLES C THOMAS • PUBLISHER
Springfield · Illinois · U.S.A.

Published and Distributed Throughout the World by
CHARLES C THOMAS · PUBLISHER
BANNERSTONE HOUSE
301-327 East Lawrence Avenue, Springfield, Illinois, U.S.A.
NATCHEZ PLANTATION HOUSE
735 North Atlantic Boulevard, Fort Lauderdale, Florida, U.S.A.

This book is protected by copyright. No
part of it may be reproduced in any manner
without written permission from the publisher.

© *1972, by* CHARLES C THOMAS · PUBLISHER
ISBN 0–398–02222–4
Library of Congress Catalog Card Number: 76-175066

With THOMAS BOOKS *careful attention is given to all details of
manufacturing and design. It is the Publisher's desire to present books
that are satisfactory as to their physical qualities and artistic possibilities
and appropriate for their particular use.* THOMAS BOOKS *will be true
to those laws of quality that assure a good name and good will.*

Printed in the United States of America
Y-2

Library
University of Texas
at San Antonio

PREFACE

Since the introduction of chlorpromazine, a large number of neuro-leptic drugs, useful in the treatment of schizophrenic patients, have been synthesized. These new drugs, with increasingly well-defined behavioral, neurophysiological and biochemical actions, have provided new means for therapeutically influencing and systematically studying schizophrenic psychopathology. Nevertheless, apart from their therapeutic impact by effectively controlling certain symptoms of schizophrenia, the question remains as to what extent these improvements have led to any fundamental breakthrough in our understanding of either schizophrenia or the schizophrenic patient.

Development of the psychopharmacological method has led to reassessment of instruments and points of reference in psychiatry. Accordingly, in this monograph the psychopharmacological approach is applied to problems related to schizophrenia and the analysis and description of changes brought about by the introduction of new drugs in schizophrenic patients. To fulfill these aims, the second chapter provides information on new drugs with "antipsychotic" properties, the third describes their effect on schizophrenic patients and the fourth chapter discusses the gradual change in our concepts of schizophrenia.

My own observations included in the manuscript were made on the schizophrenic patient population of Douglas Hospital, Verdun, and is an expansion of the Annual Hoffman-LaRoche Lecture presented at the Clarke Institute of Psychiatry in Toronto on January 15, 1971. Since the material of this monograph has not been integrated as yet in textbooks, it is hoped that both students and practitioners of psychiatry will find this new information useful.

THOMAS A. BAN

v

ACKNOWLEDGMENTS

For the permission to use tables and figures from their publications, thanks are due to the following authors, journals and publishers:

Brill, H. and Patton, R. E.: Analysis of population reduction in New York State Mental Hospitals during the first four years of large scale therapy with psychotropic drugs. *Amer. J. Psychiat., 116*: 495-509, 1959.

Cawley, R. H.: The present status of physical methods of treatment of schizophrenia. In Coppen, A. and Walk, A. (Eds.): *Recent Developments in Schizophrenia.* Ashford, Headley Brothers, 1967.

Kelly, D. H. W. and Sargent, W.: Present treatment of schizophrenia. A controlled follow-up study. *Brit. Med. J., 1*:147-150, 1965.

Klein, D. F. and Davis, J. M.: Diagnosis and Drug Treatment of Psychiatric Disorders. Baltimore, Williams & Wilkins, 1969.

Med. Letter Drugs Therap., 12(25):104, 1970.

I am particularly grateful to Doctor H. E. Lehmann for reading the first draft of this manuscript and for his valuable suggestions, and to Doctor W. Horsley Gantt for accepting this monograph in the American Lecture Series.

I am thankful to Mrs. Joan Dickie for the typing of the manuscript and for the verifying of the references, and to my wife for her assistance in the various phases of writing.

CONTENTS

SCHIZOPHRENIA
A Psychopharmacological Approach

Chapter 1

INTRODUCTION

THE psychopharmacological era began on January 19th, 1952, when chlorpromazine was given for the first time to a psychiatric patient by Hamon, Paraire and Velluz (1952) at Val-de-Grâce, the famed military hospital in Paris. From Val-de-Grâce, chlorpromazine therapy in psychiatry raced through the mental hospitals of France within the single year of 1952 (Delay and Deniker, 1952), transforming disturbed wards, reforming therapy and remodelling research (Caldwell, 1970a,b). Swiss psychiatrists introduced chlorpromazine in January, 1953 (Staehelin and Kielholz, 1953), and by the spring of 1953, the "psychopharmacological revolution" was well underway throughout continental Europe. Lehmann and Hanrahan's (1954) paper, the first American publication on chlorpromazine, appeared as early as February, 1954, in the American Medical Association's *Archives of Neurology and Psychiatry*; and one year later, the first Australian and Russian publications were also in print (Tarasov, 1955; Webb, 1955).

The basic constituent of chlorpromazine is the phenothiazine nucleus which consists of two benzol rings attached to each other by a sulfur and a nitrogen atom (Fig.1). It was synthesized on December

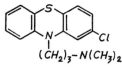

Figure 1. The structural formula of chlorpromazine.

11, 1950, by Charpentier and his collaborators (1952); released for clinical studies by May 2, 1951, upon completion of the initial pharmacological investigations by Courvoisier and her team (1953); and

3

had been first tried as an "autonomic stabilizer" to bring about a condition that Laborit (1951) described as "artificial hibernation" within the same year.

The first article on chlorpromazine appeared in *Presse Médicale* on February 13, 1952. In this, Laborit, Huguenard and Alluaume (1952) described the fundamental observation that "in doses of 50 to 100 mg intravenously, chlorpromazine does not produce loss of consciousness or a change in patient's mentality, but it does produce a slight tendency to sleep and above all an indifference to the surroundings."

In the subsequent decade, at least fifty million patients received chlorpromazine; more than ten thousand reports were published on the drug (Jarvik, 1965); and at least one hundred other psychoactive drugs were synthesized and investigated. Nevertheless, apart from these drugs' therapeutic impact, the question remains to what extent their introduction has become instrumental in elucidating biochemical, physiological, behavioral and psychological mechanisms involved in clinical psychopathological problems. While no one would doubt that the introduction of chlorpromazine and subsequently of other psychotherapeutic drugs brought about important changes by effectively controlling certain symptoms of schizophrenia, allowing the rehabilitation of many patients who appeared doomed to a lifetime of hospitalization (Hollister, 1970), the question also remains as to what extent these improvements have led to any fundamental breakthrough in our understanding of either schizophrenia or the schizophrenic patient.

Fluphenazine

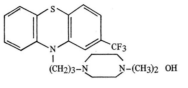

Methophenazine

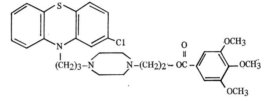

Perphenazine

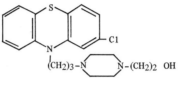

Prochlorperazine

Figure 3*b*

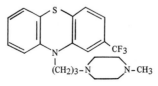

Thiopropazate

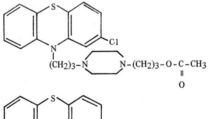

Thioproperazine

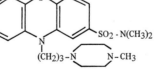

Trifluoperazine

Figure 3*c*

Mesoridazine

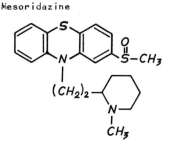

Piperacetazine

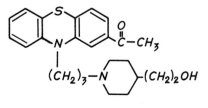

Propericiazine

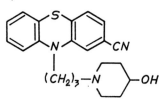

Thioridazine

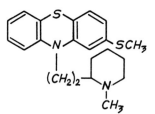

Figure 4. Structural formula of piperidylalkyl phenothiazine derivatives: mesoridazine, piperacetazine, propericiazine and thioridazine.

Chen, 1970). Whether clomacran will find a place in the treatment of schizophrenic patients remains to be seen (Fig. 6).

Rauwolfia Alkaloids and Related Drugs

The same year the unique neuroleptic properties of chlorpromazine were discovered, the active principle of the snakeroot plant (*Rauwolfia serpentina*), which had been used for centuries in India as a treatment for a variety of mental and emotional disorders, was isolated and identified as reserpine (Serpasil®) by Mueller, Schlittler and Bein (1952). The first paper on the therapeutic effects of *R serpentina* in psychiatric patients was presented by Hakim (1953), which was soon followed by Kline's (1954) historical report on the usefulness of *reserpine* in the treatment of psychotic patients in general and schizophrenic patients in particular (Ban, 1969a; Lehmann and Ban, 1970). For a while, it seemed that with reserpine the success story of chlorpromazine was being repeated. From Rockland State Hospital— Kline's research facilities — reserpine therapy in psychiatry raced through mental hospitals not only in the the United States but all over the world. Numerous other neuroleptic *Rauwolfia* alkaloids were

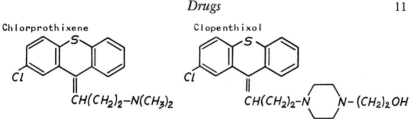

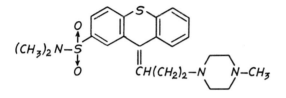

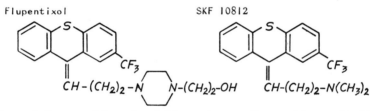

Figure 5. Structural formula of thioxanthenes: chlorprothixene, thiothixene, clopenthixol, flupentixol and SKF 10812.

isolated and employed in the treatment of psychiatric patients; among them, deserpidine and rescinnamine were clinically the most important. Although in fourteen out of twenty-six comparative studies reserpine was found to be equally effective to chlorpromazine (Klein and Davis, 1969), reserpine therapy reached an early climax because of its unreliable therapeutic activity (Kurland, 1956; Wright and Kyne, 1960), and by the 1960's its use had virtually been abandoned in the treatment of schizophrenic patients (Fig. 7).

Pharmacologically similar to but structurally different from the *Rauwolfia* alkaloids are the two clinically studied *benzoquinolizines*, tetrabenazine and benzquinamide. As with reserpine, the sedative effect of tetrabenazine in animals is accompanied by depletion of serotonin (5HT) and norepinephrine (NE) levels in the brain. In spite

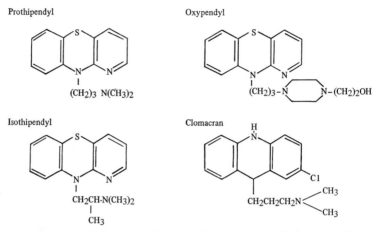

Figure 6. Structural formula of benzothiazines and acridanes: prothipendyl, oxypendyl and isothipendyl; and clomacran.

of its antipsychotic properties and proven therapeutic value (Ashcroft, MacDougall and Barker, 1961; Bertolotti and Munarini, 1961; Burckard *et al.*, 1962; Kammerer *et al.*, 1962; Lingjaerde, 1963), tetrabenazine has never been introduced into the treatment of schizophrenic patients because of its numerous side effects. The same applies to benzquinamide, a serotonin antagonist (Feldman, 1962; Overall *et al.*, 1963a; Sainz, 1963; Scriabine *et al.*, 1963; Settel, 1963) (Fig. 8).

Butyrophenone Derivatives and Related Drugs

Besides the phenothiazines, the most extensively explored neuroleptic drugs are the *butyrophenones* (Janssen, 1965). They were developed in the late 1950's by Janssen and his collaborators (1959, 1960) who in the course of systematic efforts to increase the morphine-like potency of drugs, studied a large series of 4-phenyl-piperidines related to pethidine (meperidine) which resulted in the first neuroleptic butyrophenone substance. In the subsequent ten years, haloperidol, trifluperidol, methylperidol, floropipamide, dehydrobenzperidol, benzperidol, spiroperidol and fluanisone, i.e. eight different neuroleptic butyrophenone derivatives have been clinically studied (Janssen, 1965; Pöldinger and Schmidlin, 1966), and at least another four, i.e. CI-601, chemically designated as 4-[2-(o-ethoxyphenoxy)-ethyl]amino-4'-fluorobutyrophenone monohydrochloride; AI-449, chemically 4-(4-hydroxypiperidino)-4-fluorobutyrophenone hydro-

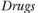

Reserpine

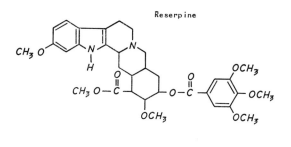

Deserpidine

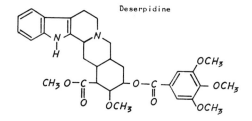

Rescinnamine

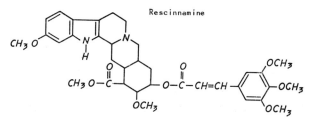

Figure 7. Structural formula of *Rauwolfia* alkaloids: reserpine, deserpidine and rescinnamine.

chloride; AL-1021, chemically 1-3-(4-fluorobenzoyl)propyl-4-peri-dyl N-isopropyl carbonate; and AHR-1900, chemically 4' fluoro-4-[3-(o-methoxy-phenoxy)-1-pyrrolidinyl], have been systematically investigated (Ban, 1962, 1964, 1969b; Ban and Lehmann, 1967, Ban and Stonehill, 1964; Gallant and Bishop, 1969; Gallant, Bishop and Guerrero-Figueroa, 1968; Lehmann and Ban, 1964a; Lehmann *et al.*, 1964; Sugerman, 1968; Sugerman, Herrmann and O'Hara, 1970; Villeneuve *et al.*, 1970; Warnes, Lee and Ban, 1964). It is interesting to note that of this large variety of drugs, only haloperidol has been

Tetrabenazine

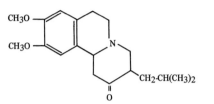

Benzquinamide

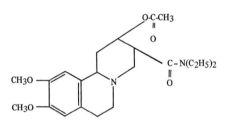

Figure 8. Structural formula of benzoquinolizines: tetrabenazine and benzquinamide.

used in the United States and Canada in the treatment of schizophrenic patients (Fig. 9).

Another series of neuroleptics structurally and pharmacologically related to the butyrophenones are the *diphenylbutylpiperidines* (Janssen *et al.*, 1968). From this group, pimozide, chemically designated as 1-[[1-[4,4-bis(p-fluorophenyl)butyl]-4-piperidyl]]-2 benzimidazolone; and fluspirilene, a long-acting parenteral preparation chemically designated as 8-[4,4-bis-(p-fluorophenyl)-butyl]-1- phenyl-1,3,8 triazaspiro[4,5] decan-4-on, have been clinically investigated (Bonbon *et al.*, 1968; Brugmans, 1968; Chouinard *et al.*, 1970; Chouinard, Lehmann and Ban, 1970; Haase *et al.*, 1968; Madalena, 1969; Sterkmans, Brugmans and Gevers, 1968, 1969) (Fig. 10).

Other Drug Groups

There are at least two other classes of neuroleptic drugs under clinical investigation—the *phenylpiperazines* (oxypertine and C1-383 chemically designated as 4-[o-propylthiophenyl]-1-piperazinepentanol) and the *indolic derivatives* (molindone) (Claghorn, 1969; Ramsey *et al.*, 1970a, b; Shelton, Prusmack and Hollister, 1968; Simpson and Krakov, 1968; Skarbek and Hill, 1967; Skarbek and Jacobsen, 1965; Sugerman and Herrmann, 1967) (Fig. 11).

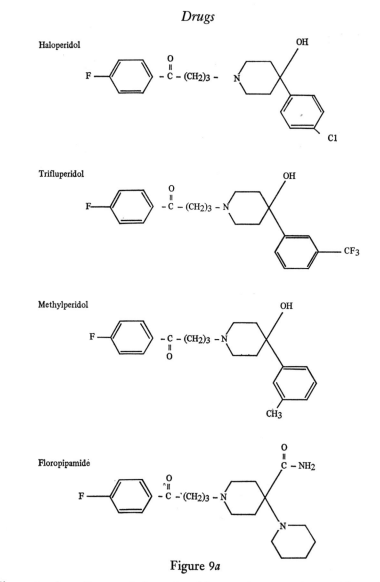

Haloperidol

Trifluperidol

Methylperidol

Floropipamidė

Figure 9*a*

Figure 9*a, b, c.* Structural formula of butyrophenones: haloperidol, triflu-peridol, methylperidol, floropipamide, dehydrobenzperidol, benzperidol, spi-roperidol, fluanisone, CI-601, AI-449, AL-1021 and AHR-1900.

Dehydrobenzperidol

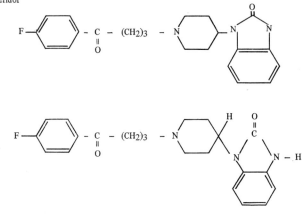

Benzperidol

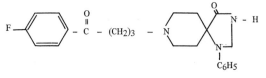

Spiroperidol

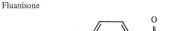

Fluanisone

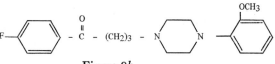

Figure 9*b*

CLINICAL EFFECTS

General Results

Psychiatric opinion is notoriously capricious and usually divided on many issues. Yet when it comes to neuroleptic drugs, there is an impressive consensus of opinion (Cawley, 1967). Thus, for example, Bannister, Salmon and Leiberman (1964) found the highest concordance of all diagnosis-treatment relationships in psychiatry between the diagnosis of schizophrenia and treatment with phenothiazines. Furthermore, in the same study, Willis and Bannister (1965) found that of 205 senior psychiatrists in England, 96 percent used phenothiazines and/or other neuroleptic drugs in the treatment of schizophrenic patients.

Cl - 601

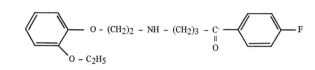

Al - 449

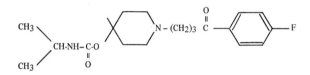

AL - 1021

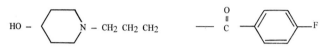

AHR - 1900

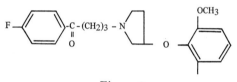

Figure 9c

Specific Results

Are Neuroleptics Effective?

However obvious it seems today, the superiority of therapeutically employed neuroleptics to placebo, i.e. the simple fact that neuroleptics are effective, had to be established, and it took approximately eight years from the first psychiatric application of chlorpromazine to provide sufficient evidence that they do have a therapeutic action.

In the United States Veterans Administration (VA) Collaborative Studies, first the superiority of chlorpromazine and promazine over an active (phenobarbital) and an inactive placebo was demonstrated in chronic schizophrenics; and later, the superiority of chlorproma-

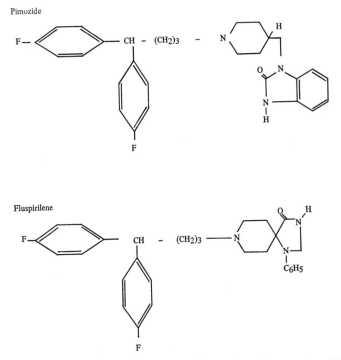

Figure 10. Structural formula of diphenylbutylpiperidines: pimozide and fluspirilene.

zine, mepazine,* perphenazine, prochlorperazine, and trifluoperazine over an active placebo was also shown in newly admitted schizophrenic patients (Casey *et al.*, 1960a, b).

Findings in the VA Collaborative Studies were supported by Adelson and Epstein (1962) and in the National Institute of Mental Health (NIMH) Collaborative Studies (1964). In the former, chlorpromazine, perphenazine, prochlorperazine and triflupromazine were found to be superior to both an active and inactive placebo in chronic schizophrenics; and in the latter, chlorpromazine, fluphenazine and thioridazine were found to be superior to an inactive placebo in acute schizophrenic patients (Table II).

Of the clinically used nonphenothiazine neuroleptics, the *Rauwolfia* alkaloid reserpine was shown to be superior to placebo in twenty (out of 29) clinical studies (Klein and Davies, 1969); the butyro-

*Mepazine was taken off the market because of toxic effects.

Oxypertine

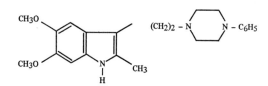

Cl - 383

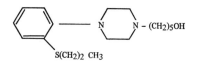

Molindone

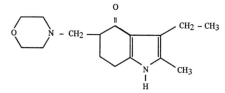

Figure 11. Structural formula of phenylpiperazines and indolic derivatives: oxypertine and CI-383; and molindone.

TABLE II

EARLY STUDIES IN WHICH SUPERIORITY OF NEUROLEPTICS
OVER PLACEBO WAS DEMONSTRATED

Studies	In Acute Patients (Drugs)	In Chronic Patients (Drugs)
I. U.S. Veterans Administration Collaborative Studies (Casey et al., 1960a).		chlorpromazine promazine
II. U.S. Veterans Administration Collaborative Studies (Casey et al., 1960b).	chlorpromazine mepazine perphenazine prochlorperazine trifluoperazine	
III. Adelson and Epstein (1962).		chlorpromazine perphenazine prochlorperazine triflupromazine
IV. N.I.M.H. Collaborative Studies Group (1964).	chlorpromazine fluphenazine thioridazine	

TABLE III

NUMBER OF STUDIES IN WHICH DRUG WAS MORE EFFECTIVE
THAN PLACEBO*

Drug	No. of Studies Reviewed in which Drug was	
	More Effective than Placebo	Equal to Placebo
Phenothiazines:		
Chlorpromazine	50	11
Triflupromazine	8	1
Perphenazine	5	0
Prochlorperazine	7	2
Trifluoperazine	16	2
Fluphenazine	9	0
Thioridazine	6	1
Total Phenothiazines:	101	17
Rauwolfia Alkaloids:		
Reserpine	20	9

*Klein and Davis, 1969.

phenone haloperidol was superior in at least five (Azima, Durost and
Arthurs, 1960; Garry and Leonard, 1962; Okasha and Twefik, 1964;
Simpson, Angus and Edwards, 1967; Sugerman, Williams and Adlerstein, 1964); the thioxanthene derivative chlorprothixene was also
superior in at least five (Cappelen and Monrad, 1961; Felger, 1965;
Fincle and Johnson, 1965; Karn, Mead and Fishman, 1961; Scanlan
and May, 1963); and thiothixene was superior in at least one (Sterlin, Oliveros and Ban, 1968).

In their review on controlled studies, Cole, Goldberg and Davis
(1966) gave an account of a large number of psychoactive phenothiazines (chlorpromazine, fluphenazine, thioridazine, trifluperazine, prochlorperazine and perphenazine) which were found to be
more effective than placebo. Placebo equaled the active phenothiazine
preparation in only twenty-four out of ninety-five studies, while in
seventy-one it was definitely inferior to the various neuroleptic drugs.
Small patient samples, low drug dosage and/or short treatment duration were common characteristics of the studies in which the superiority of the active substance could not be shown. Similar findings
were reported in Klein and Davis's (1969) survey in which placebo
equaled the active phenothiazine preparation in only 17 out of 118

TABLE IV

DOSE REGIMES OF STUDIES IN WHICH CHLORPROMAZINE WAS
MORE EFFECTIVE THAN PLACEBO AND OF STUDIES IN WHICH
CHLORPROMAZINE WAS NOT MORE EFFECTIVE THAN PLACEBO*

Chlorpromazine mg/day	More Effective than Placebo in No. of Studies	Equal to Placebo in No. of Studies
< 300	16	9
301-400	7	1
401-500	4	1
501-800	14	0
> 800	9	0

*Klein and Davis, 1969.

studies, while in 101 it was definitely inferior to the various (chlor-promazine, triflupromazine, perphenazine, prochlorperazine, trifluo-perazine, fluphenazine and thioridazine) neuroleptic drugs (Table III). They suggested that the relatively large number of studies—eleven out of sixty-one—in which chlorpromazine was found to be equal and not superior in its therapeutic efficacy to placebo occurred during initial clinical trials when adequate dose levels had not yet been determined and improvement measures were crude. Most studies which found chlorpromazine ineffective did, in fact, use very small doses, i.e. 300 mg/day or less. On the other hand, in all the studies in which it was administered in adequate dosages, i.e. 500 mg/day or more, chlorpromazine was found to be more effective than placebo (Table IV).

While it took approximately eight years to demonstrate in an acceptable manner that neuroleptics do work, by now there has been abundant evidence repeatedly given that neuroleptics are effective drugs in the treatment of schizophrenic patients (Table V).

Is One Neuroleptic Better than the Other?

With the rapidly growing number of clinically used neuroleptics synthesized with the purpose of modifying, enhancing and superseding the therapeutic effects of chlorpromazine and eliminate its undesired reactions, it becomes increasingly important that every new neuroleptic should have a better therapeutic index than chlorpromazine or any of the other clinically used neuroleptic drugs. Of course a neuroleptic with a better therapeutic index fulfills this purpose,

TABLE V

NEUROLEPTICS AVAILABLE IN THE UNITED STATES AND / OR
IN CANADA IN ESTIMATED EQUIVALENT DOSES

Generic Names	Estimated Equivalent Dose
Chlorpromazine	100
Methotrimeprazine	75
Promazine	100
Triflupromazine	25
Acetophenazine	20
Butaperazine	10
Carphenazine	25
Fluphenazine	2
Perphenazine	10
Prochlorperazine	15
Thiopropazate	10
Thioproperazine	5
Trifluoperazine	5
Mesoridazine	75
Piperacetazine	10
Propericiazine	15
Thioridazine	100
Chlorprothixene	100
Thiothixene	2
Reserpine	2
Haloperidol	2

while a neuroleptic with a lower or even equal therapeutic index contributes to a chaotic therapeutic situation, which is disadvantageous to the schizophrenic patient.

For some time it has been noted that differences among the clinically used neuroleptics are small or practically nil, at least insofar as overall therapeutic efficacy is concerned. The first supporting evidence for this rather widely held view, however, was only given in 1966 by Cole, Goldberg and Davis. In none of the studies they reviewed were any of the phenothiazine drugs superior in overall therapeutic efficacy to chlorpromazine, but in some of the studies promazine (Casey *et al.*, 1960a; Kurland *et al.*, 1962) and mepazine (Casey *et al.*, 1960b) were significantly less effective. Promazine and mepazine were also shown to be inferior in their therapeutic efficacy to perphenazine, prochlorperazine, triflupromazine, fluphenazine and thioridazine (Casey *et al.*, 1960a; Klein and Davis, 1969; Kurland *et al.*, 1962), while the latter drugs were found to be equal, but not superior, in their therapeutic effectiveness to each other and also to chlorpromazine.

Similarly, there was no consistent evidence that any of the clinically used *Rauwolfia* alkaloid (reserpine), butyrophenone (haloperidol) or thioxanthene (chlorprothixene and thiothixene) preparations were superior to chlorpromazine or to any of the other neuroleptic phenothiazines (Bishop, Fulmer and Gallant, 1966; Hollister *et al.*, 1962; Lasky *et al.*, 1962; Lehmann *et al.*, 1964; Sterlin, Oliveros and Ban, 1968; Sterlin *et al.*, 1970). On the other hand, in some of the studies reserpine was found to be inferior in its therapeutic efficacy to chlorpromazine and also to fluphenazine and thioridazine (Lasky *et al.*, 1962; Simon *et al.*, 1958).

While the effort to supersede the therapeutic effects of chlorpromazine has failed, there are indications that the newer neuroleptics may produce less adverse effects. A recent review lists fourteen undesired reactions with various classes of neuroleptic drugs (*Medical Letter*, 1970). Of these, twelve to thirteen were encountered with phenothiazines, ten with thioxanthenes and eight with butyrophenones (Table VI).

Do Neuroleptics Differ in their Action?

The relatively limited decrease in toxicity without a substantial increase in therapeutic efficacy does not justify the rather large number of clinically available neuroleptics. Nevertheless, if the new neuroleptics would qualitatively differ in their therapeutic action from the older ones in general or chlorpromazine in particular, this alone would justify their existence.

It was a common clinical contention for some time that hyperactive patients responded best to phenothiazine treatment, whereas withdrawn patients deteriorated on the same treatment regime. It was also believed that the more sedative phenothiazines, such as chlorpromazine, methotrimeprazine or thioridazine, were preferable for patients with agitation, and the less sedative drugs, such as trifluoperazine, prochlorperazine and perphenazine, were preferable for patients with symptoms of withdrawal and retardation. Supporting data for

TABLE VI

NATURE OF ADVERSE REACTIONS TO VARIOUS GROUPS OF NEUROLEPTICS*

	Phenothiazines				
	Aminoalkyls	Piperazinylalkyls	Piperidylalkyls	Butyrophenones	Thioxanthenes
Oversedation	+++	-	+++	-	+++
Parkinson's Syndrome	++	++	++	+++	++
Akathisia	+++	+++	+++	++++	++
Dystonic reactions	++	+++	++	+++	++++
Anticholinergic effects	+++	+++	++	-	++
Postural hypotension	+++	+	+++	+	++
Inhibition of ejaculation	++	++	-	-	-
Lenticular pigmentation	+	+	++	-	-
Pigmentary retinopathy	-	-	-	-	-
Allergic skin reaction	++	+	++	-	++
Photosensitivity reaction	++	+	+++	++	+
ECG abnormalities	+	+	++	-	-
Cholestatic jaundice	++	+++	+++	++	++
Blood dyscrasias	++		++	++	++

* *Medical Letter*, 1970.
ECG abnormalities were added to the effects included in *Medical Letter*.
+++, frequent
++, occasional
+, rare

this contention were obtained from the answers to a questionnaire from fifty-four consultant psychiatrists working in mental hospitals, teaching hospitals and academic units. They were asked to indicate their preference in the prescription of eleven phenothiazines (chlorpromazine, methotrimeprazine, promazine and triflupromazine; thioridazine; and fluphenazine, perphenazine, prochlorperazine, thiopropazate, trifluoperazine and trifluoproperazine) for thirteen syndromes of psychiatric illness. Among the syndromes, those which applied to the treatment of schizophrenia were specified in the questionnaire as syndromes dominated (a) by apathy and inertia, (b) by overactive behavior, and (c) by paranoid features. The greatest consensus regarding treatment showed chlorpromazine as the treatment of choice for overactive behavior, trifluoperazine as the treatment of choice for apathy and inertia, and both chlorpromazine and trifluoperazine as substantially useful in paranoid syndromes. Thioridazine and perphenazine were the next most fashionable drugs, and the other seven phenothiazines were little used (Cawley, 1967) (Fig. 12).

However disappointing it may be, these findings were contradicted by well-designed and appropriately conducted studies. Marks (1963), using data from a large cooperative study, did not find that patients with excitement responded better to the more sedative-type phenothiazines such as chlorpromazine or that patients who were withdrawn responded better to the more activating phenothiazines such as perphenazine. Similarly, Platz, Klett and Caffey (1967) in a 28-week study with 330 patients, dividing patients into the older categories of "hyperdynamic" and "hypodynamic" based on the degree of their activity and somatization, failed to reveal any preferential action of chlorpromazine in the "hyperdynamic" and of carphenazine and trifluperazine in the "hypodynamic" type of patient. Analysis of covariance on the seventeen rating scales and one global measure showed no significant differences among the three drug groups for the 24-weeks treatment period.

All attempts to reveal differential clinical effects among neuroleptics fall short of verification to date. For example, Overall *et al.* (1963b), through computer analysis of initial ratings on the Brief Psychiatric Rating Scale (BPRS) (using pattern probability models based on presenting signs and symptoms), divided ninety-eight schizophrenics into three subtypes—"paranoid," "core" and "depressed."

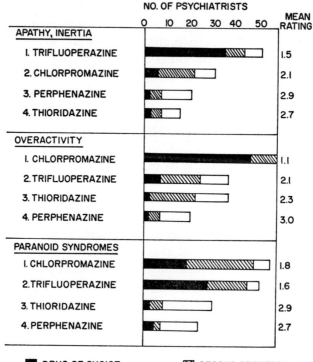

Figure 12. Use of phenothiazines for various psychopathological symptoms in schizophrenia by psychiatrists (Cawley, 1967).

They found that all three schizophrenic subtypes responded equally to perphenazine, but paranoid patients responded more favorably to acetophenazine. Cross-validation of this study, however, was not successful (Hollister *et al.*, 1967). Instead, the replication study indicated that paranoid patients in general tended to respond somewhat better than the other types. In another study, Klett and Moseley (1965) seemed to succeed in predicting treatment—chlorpromazine or fluphenazine—outcome by using multiple correlations with pretreatment symptoms. When tested against actual results, the interactions were significant. Their predictive equations, however, did not hold up in a cross-validation attempt with a second patient sample (Galbrecht and Klett, 1968). In the NIMH Collaborative Study (NIMH-PRB 1967) 480 acutely ill schizophrenic patients were divided into four types—"core," "paranoid," "bizarre" and "depressive"—and the actions of three phenothiazines, chlorpromazine, acetophenazine and fluphenazine, were compared in each. It was found that chlorpromazine was most efficacious for "core," acetophenazine for "bizarre" and "depressive" and fluphenazine for "depressive" types of patients. In another study, the same group tried to predict treatment outcome by using regression equations based on pretreatment symptoms (Goldberg *et al.*, 1967). According to them, the chlorpromazine improver has a greater number of core symptoms of schizophrenia than those who improve on other drugs, while the acetophenazine improver seems to show paranoid excitement with social participation; the fluphenazine improver is irritable, indifferent, with poor social participation, poor self care and has feelings of unreality; and the thioridazine improver is agitated, sad, manifests pressured speech and also has feelings of unreality. Nevertheless, in a later review, Goldberg (1968), one of the principal investigators in these studies, concluded that the evidence for a differential action of neuroleptic drugs was highly inconclusive. This state of affairs has not changed since.

After the introduction of chlorpromazine, it was hoped that it would bring about a new psychopharmacological era in psychiatry in which drugs, with well-defined behavioral, neurophysiological and biochemical actions would be used not only in treatment but also in the systematic study of psychopathological conditions. These expectations have not been fulfilled to date. Instead, we have a confoundingly large number of neuroleptics with more or less equal overall therapeutic efficacy but without any clearly defined differential therapeutic indications.

Chapter 3

PATIENTS

OVERALL EFFECTS

IN SPITE of all its limitations, the treatment of choice today for schizophrenia is pharmacotherapy. According to Lehmann (1965), "no other single therapeutic procedure can compete with it in terms of rapid effectiveness, sustained action, general availability and ease of application." Furthermore, "it compares favorably with other therapies as far as incidence of side effects, complications and serious risks are concerned." While the rate of spontaneous recovery from schizophrenia has been determined to be about 15 to 25 percent, modern pharmacotherapy had by 1963 resulted in a social recovery rate between 50 to 60 percent for patients who had been ill for less than three years (Pearson, 1963) and a discharge rate of 75 to 80 percent for all acute hospitalized patients within a year and of more than 50 percent within six months (Lehmann, 1966). Reports from several countries have indicated that as a result of neuroleptics, (a) the annual increase of admissions to psychiatric beds has been reduced or terminated, (b) the average duration of hospital stay has been shortened, (c) the number of discharges has greatly increased and (d) the number of patients followed up in a state of social remission has increased. In other instances, however, it has been shown that the percentage of schizophrenics admitted to hospital or remaining in residence has been unaltered in the neuroleptic era (Chanoit *et al.*, 1970).

Neuroleptics and the Natural Course of Schizophrenia

The first information on the natural course of schizophrenia dates back to Kraepelin (1896), who described dementia praecox as a disease which is always progressive and particularly with regard to emotional deterioration. In a few cases, however, the process may come to a standstill and some of the symptoms may even disappear, but far more commonly the outcome is deep deterioration. Accordingly, his figures for a group of inpatients at the Heidelberg Hospital showed that of the 12.6 percent who had a complete remission first, 8.5 percent relapsed three to six years later; and only 4.1 percent remained well. The figure of 12.6 percent could be raised to 13.3 percent by adding to it all the cases with only a mild defect and to 17 percent by extending it with all the cases who could live a more or less socially adjusted life independent of the degree of defect (Hoenig, 1967). On the other hand, 70 percent of Kraepelin's dementia praecox patients deeply deteriorated.

The three crucial figures of Kraepelin (1896, 1910) on the natural course of schizophrenia are full recovery, 4.1 percent; social remission, 17 percent; and deterioration, 70 percent. It is interesting to note the little variation in these figures during the prepsychopharmacological era. Thus, Evensen (1904) in his first study reported on 15 percent social remissions (somewhat less than Kraepelin's) and 60 percent deep deterioration (also somewhat less than Kraepelin's). His sample consisted of male schizophrenics less than twenty-six years old first admitted to the Gastaud Hospital between 1887 and 1896; and his evaluation was based on a five- to fifteen-year follow-up. After a similar follow-up period on a sample of 815 schizophrenic patients discharged from the Gastaud Hospital between 1915 and 1929, Evensen (1936) found that 23 percent of the patients were self-supportive or in social remission. This was a modest improvement to his own and also to Kraepelin's earlier findings.* Similar to Kraepelin's are Langfeldt's (1937) figures based on a seven- to thirteen-year follow-up study on 100 schizophrenic patients. In his sample, 66 percent were uncured or worse (just 4 percent less than in Kraepelin's) and 17 percent were completely recovered. When this 17 percent was broken down further, however, 14 percent consisted of patients with a quite atypical—so-called schizophreniform—clinical picture. Taking off the 14 percent of patients with schizophreniform

---

*Admissions to the Gastaud Hospital from 1938 to 1950 have been followed up (by Ödegard, 1968) and it was noted that social remissions further increased (from 23 percent) to 35 percent. The follow-up of admission cohorts after 1950 is not completed, but preliminary results show a further rise to 51 percent.

TABLE VII

SOCIAL REMISSION OF SCHIZOPHRENIC PATIENTS DURING
THE PERIOD 1896 TO 1966

	Full Recovery %	*Social Remission* %	*Deterioration* %
Kraepelin (1896)	4.1	17.0	70.0
Evensen (1904)		15.0	60.0
Evensen (1935)		23.0	
Langfeldt (1937)	17.0 (14+3)		66.0
Achté (1961)		65.0	
Simon (1965)		20.0	80.0 (30+50)
Hoenig & Hamilton (1966)		55.0	

psychosis leaves 3 percent full recoveries, which is only slightly less than Kraepelin's figure (Hoenig, 1967).

It is unfortunate that there are no real comparative data available on the basis of which one could assess the effect of neuroleptics on the natural course of schizophrenia. Reports from the neuroleptic era have yielded controversial findings. In an eight-year follow-up study with eighty patients treated with chlorpromazine or reserpine, Simon *et al.* (1965) found that only 20 percent improved in their psychiatric adjustment and work record; nearly 50 percent were rated as worse (deteriorated); and 30 percent as unchanged. These findings did not differ essentially from those in the prepsychopharmacological era. In variance with these findings are the results of Hoenig and Hamilton (1966), whose follow-up study included sixty-two schizophrenic patients. At the end of a four-year follow-up period, they found 27.5 percent of the patients symptom-free, another 27.5 percent much improved (i.e. 55 percent social remission), 16.5 percent unchanged and 9.7 percent dead. (Information could not be obtained for the remaining 19 percent.) These figures compare very favorably to previous findings, but as Hoenig (1967) suggests, the change was only partly due to the drugs. In fact, social recovery in Achté's (1961) four-year follow-up study on patients admitted between 1953 to 1955, i.e., during the prepsychopharmacological era, was somewhat higher, 65 percent, than in Hoenig and Hamilton's (1966) report (Table VII).

Neuroleptics and Psychiatric Hospitalization
Population Changes in Hospitals

Much more convincing than the action on the natural course of schizophrenia are the effects of neuroleptics on population changes in mental hospitals. This was elegantly demonstrated by Brill and Patton in three consecutive studies (1957, 1959, 1962).

According to Brill and Patton's reports in 1955, the resident population of New York state's mental hospitals had reached an all-time high of 93,600 as a result of the continuation of a long-term trend that had doubled the mental hospital cases since 1929. Then in 1955 and 1956, this upward trend was abruptly reversed. The drop in resident population continued with an increasing tendency for at least another three years (Fig. 13) and gained significance from the fact that it was coincidental with the introduction of neuroleptic drugs in the therapy of hospitalized patients (Fig. 14).

Comparing the hospital population of March 31, 1955, with that of March 31, 1958, i.e. after three years of pharmacological treatment, Brill and Patton (1959) found an overall reduction of 2123 patients. The largest reduction, 2112 patients, was seen in the schizophrenic group.

Further analysis revealed that the number of patients hospitalized for ten years or longer, in spite of neuroleptics, had actually in-

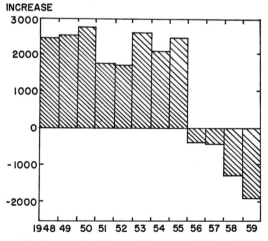

Figure 13. Annual changes in the resident population of New York State mental hospitals from 1948 to 1959 (Brill and Patton, 1959).

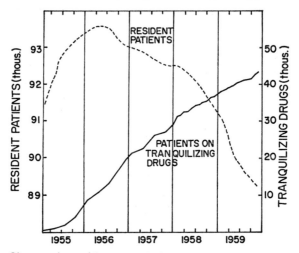

Figure 14. Changes in resident population and changes in number of patients on neuroleptics in New York State mental hospitals from 1955 to 1959
(Brill and Patton, 1959).

creased; and while the number of patients hospitalized over a five-
to nine-year period did not decrease, it had ceased to grow. On the
other hand, the two- to four-year group had fallen by 1463 patients,
and the one- to two-year group had diminished by 27 percent.
Nevertheless, the reduction in patients hospitalized for less than 1
year was less than 8 percent (Fig. 15). The fact that the greatest
reduction in the schizophrenic population occurred in patients hospitalized longer than one but less than five years indicates that the
most significant action of neuroleptics is not in the increased speed of
therapy but in the prevention of chronicity.

Duration of Hospital Stay

However impressive the fall in hospitalized schizophrenic population is, it is frequently argued that the decreasing tendency in duration of hospital stay had commenced prior to the introduction of
neuroleptic drugs.

One of the best expositions of the decreasing tendency in hospital
stay prior to the psychopharmacological era is Stern's (1970), who
analyzed the stay of patients in the Central Hospital at Warwick over
almost a 100-year period. While the duration of stay in this hospital
did not show significant variation from 1853 to 1932, he recognized

central
Hospital
at Warwick
N.York

Poster
Board

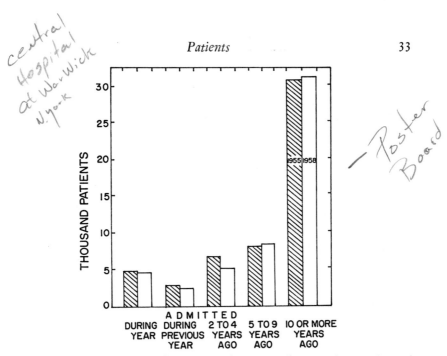

Figure 15. Reduction in patient population according to the number of years spent in hospital (Brill and Patton, 1959).

that within two years after the introduction of the Mental Treatment Act in 1930, which allowed the admission of voluntary and temporary patients, a steady decrease in the hospital stay of patients has commenced. Consequently, by 1954 discharge rate reached 84 percent from the steady 50 percent during the 1853 to 1932 period.

There are a number of other studies in which the decrease of hospital stay has been demonstrated long preceding the psychopharmacological era. Shepherd (1957) compared two groups of schizophrenics admitted to a mental hospital in the 1931 to 1933 and in the 1945 to 1947 periods. He followed them for five years and found that the 1945 to 1947 group spent considerably less time in hospital than did the 1931 to 1933 group, i.e. 39.24 months and 45.14 months respectively. Furthermore, 10 percent more patients were discharged from the later group than from the earlier one. Essentially similar findings were reported by Freyhan (1955). He compared 100 admissions in 1920 with a comparable group in 1940 and found that 65 percent of the earlier group and only 42 percent of the later group remained in hospital during the entire thirteen-year follow-up period. In Freyhan's study, twice as many patients had been discharged from the later group than from the earlier. Further substantiation of the decreasing tendency in hospitalization prior to the introduction of neuroleptics was given by Achté (1961). He took all schizophrenic patients admitted to mental hospitals in Finland between 1933 to 1935 and compared them with those admitted between 1953 to 1955. He found that in the 1933 to 1935 group, 36 percent of the patients remained permanently hospitalized over the four-year follow-up period, while in the 1953 to 1955 group, this figure was decreased to a mere 5 percent. As in Freyhan's (1955) study, twice as many patients had been discharged from the later group than from the earlier.

With the introduction of neuroleptics, the decreasing trend in hospital stays continued. This was clearly demonstrated by Hobbs, Wanklin and Ladd (1965) with three groups of patients from different time periods. They found that of the first, 1940 to 1942, group, 72.6 percent of patients were discharged; from the second, 1950 to 1952, 81.3 percent were discharged; while from the third, 1956 to 1958, 94 percent were discharged. This third group represented the psychopharmacological era. Similar results were reported by Kelly and Sargant (1965), who found that from a phenothiazine-treated group of patients, only 7 percent stayed in hospital two years after admission, in contrast to a group of patients from the prepsychopharmacological era from which 31 percent stayed in hospital two years after admission. They also revealed that the average length of hospital stay decreased from 10.7 weeks to 6.7 weeks after the introduction of neuroleptics.* Whether this further decrease in hospital stays in the psychopharmacological era is the tailend of a "historical" trend or a drug-dependent phenomenon remains a moot question.

It is commonly believed that one of the characteristics of the psychopharmacological era is the revolving door, i.e. an increase in the number of admissions parallel with the increase in the number of discharges. In New York state, for example, first admissions rose about 17 percent between 1955 and 1960, and readmissions increased by almost 50 percent (Brill and Patton, 1962). Increase in readmissions, however, has been concomitant with the decreasing trend in hos-

---

*In Battegay and Gehring's (1968) report, the corresponding figures for average duration of hospital stay were 142 days in 1952 and 92 days in 1962.

pital stay in both the prepsychopharmacological era and psycho-pharmacological era (Shepherd, 1957; Brill and Patton, 1962; Auch, 1963). In fact, at least in one of the studies (Hobbs, Wanklin and Ladd, 1965) readmissions increased with the increased discharges from the 1940 to 1942 to the 1950 to 1952 periods, i.e. before the introduction of neuroleptic treatment, but decreased to the 1940 to 1942 levels, in spite of the further increase in discharges, during the psychopharmacological era.

More recently, there are indications that the prognosis, or rather the duration of hospital stay of the readmitted schizophrenic patient is different in the psychopharmacological era than in the period prior to the introduction of neuroleptic drugs. Pritchard (1967) compared two groups of schizophrenic patients, one from the prepsychophar-macological (1952-1953) and the other from the psychopharmaco-logical (1956-1957) era. Although the short-term outcome of the group admitted during the neuroleptic era was better than that of the other group, the long-term prognosis in terms of readmission rate was similar for the two groups. The duration of stay of readmitted pa-tients, however, was shorter in the later than in the earlier group. The finding that the duration of hospitalization specifically decreased in the psychopharmacological era was supported by Ödegard (1967). He followed three separate groups, 1930-1939, 1945-1948 and 1955-1958, over a four-year period and found that while there was a marked increase in discharge rate for first admissions from 1936-1939 to 1945-1948, the chances of being discharged for readmitted patients decreased from the first to the second period. On the other hand, from 1945-1948 to 1955-1958, discharge rates continued to rise, but in the 1955-1958 group, readmissions had the same chances for discharge as had first admissions. This improved prognosis of the readmitted patients—and not the revolving door—seems to be the important and differential characteristic of the psychopharmacolog-ical era.

Prevention of Hospitalization

Another factor with a possible role in the reduction of inpatient populations is prevention of hospitalization.

The effect of neuroleptics in the prevention of hospitalization was studied in a series of systematic studies by Engelhardt and his collaborators (1960, 1963, 1964, 1967, 1970). Their schizophrenic population was drawn from a free public clinic in New York and though essentially chronic, the patients varied considerably in length of previous hospitalizations. In fact, approximately 50 percent of the patients had maintained an essentially ambulatory status prior to clinical admission. Upon admission to the project, patients were randomly assigned to three different treatment regimes, i.e., chlorpromazine, promazine or placebo, administered under double-blind conditions, and were maintained on the same medication during the entire experimental period.

The results of this study strikingly demonstrated the effectiveness of psychoactive drugs in the prevention of hospitalization of schizophrenic patients. During the first eighteen months, 28.6 percent of the fifty-six placebo-treated patients had been hospitalized as opposed to the 4.8 percent of the sixty-two chlorpromazine treated ($p < 0.001$) patients. (The hospitalization rate with promazine treatment, 18.2 percent, fell in between.) The overall hospitalization rate for the entire sample of 173 patients was 16.7 percent. Three years later, in 1963, reexamination of hospitalization rates on 445 consecutive admissions showed considerably less favorable findings. Of the 142 patients treated with placebo, 29.6 percent were hospitalized, essentially the same figure as that obtained in 1960. However, of 153 patients treated with chlorpromazine, 19.0 percent needed hospitalization, a figure substantially higher than that obtained in 1960. (The hospitalization rate under promazine treatment, 28.0 percent, again fell in between.) The difference between chlorpromazine and placebo-treated patients still remained statistically significant ($p < 0.05$), but it was considerably less impressive in 1963 than in 1960. The overall hospitalization rate for the entire sample of 445 patients was 25.4 percent, a considerable rise when compared with that reported in 1960. Since the rise in hospitalization rate was considered to be due to differences in length of therapy, after patients had an additional thirty-five months of treatment exposure, Engelhardt *et al.* (1967) reexamined the hospitalization rates in the three drug groups. A statistical comparison of the cumulative hospitalization rates for successive periods of treatment exposure showed that after twelve months of treatment, hospitalization rates for chlorpromazine- (15.1 percent) and promazine- (19.7 percent) treated patients were significantly lower (p < 0.001 and p < 0.01 respectively) than for placebo-treated patients. By fifteen months, the hospitalization rate for promazine-treated patients (23.7 percent) became statistically comparable to the hospitalization rate of placebo-treated patients (29.6 percent), whereas even after forty-eight months, hospitalization rate for chlorpromazine-treated patients (19.7 percent) remained significantly lower (p < 0.01) than hospitalization rate for placebo- (29.6 percent) treated patients. Another important observation in this study was that only a small subgroup of approximately 30 percent of the entire population needed hospitalization (or approximately 70 percent did *not need* hospitalization) over the six-year experimental period. The fact that in Hoenig and Hamilton's (1966) sample in Manchester (UK), only 14.5 percent of the schizophrenic patients were maintained without hospitalization over an even shorter time period indicates that the rate of hospitalization is both a social- and a drug-dependent phenomenon.

There is sufficient evidence to suggest that maintenance neuroleptic treatment has a definite effect on prevention of rehospitalization. Klein and Davis (1969) list at least nineteen studies in which rehospitalization followed in three to six months the discontinuation or dose reduction of neuroleptic drugs. In collaboration with Doctors St. Laurent and Cahn (1962), we demonstrated in an aftercare clinic setting that discontinuation or decrease in the dosage of prochlorperazine resulted in exacerbation of schizophrenic symptoms, which in most cases responded promptly to resumption of maintenance therapy or to an increase of dosage. These results were similar to those of Gross *et al.* (1960) who found that during the first four months in aftercare, 42 percent of those outpatients whose neuroleptic medication had been replaced for a placebo or reduced in dosage relapsed. Within six months, relapse rate in patients on a decreased dosage or placebo was more than three times higher (51 percent) than in patients whose phenothiazine medication was continued (13 percent). There was also a threefold increase in relapse rate among patients whose neuroleptic medication was discontinued or reduced in dosage, in comparison to those patients whose medication had not been decreased, in Gantz and Birkett's (1965) double-blind, placebo-controlled clinical study.

Brill and Patton (1962) in their clinical-statistical analysis of population changes in New York state mental hospitals after the introduction of psychotropic drugs showed that simultaneous with the fall of resident population there was an approximately 50 percent increase in readmissions during the 1955 to 1960 period. Since maintenance treatment for schizophrenic patients was consistently employed only in the 1960's, it would be instructive to compare readmission rates between 1955 to 1960 and 1965 to 1970.

Neuroleptics in the Psychiatric Hospital

Behavioral Effects

After the introduction of neuroleptic drugs, positive behavioral effects on schizophrenic patients were immediately noted in psychiatric hospitals. The beneficial behavioral effects of neuroleptics were substantiated by Brill and Patton (1959), who were able to demonstrate that reduction in the use of restraint and seclusion was one of the earliest effects of the new drugs and the one which has been most consistent (Fig 16). With the rapid increase in the number of patients treated with neuroleptic drugs, there was a rapid decrease in the need of restraint, which, however, reached a plateau by 1959 at one-eighth of the original level. It was assumed that the behavioral

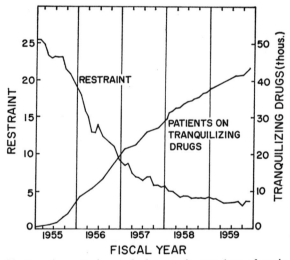

Figure 16. Changes in restraint and changes in number of patients on neuroleptics in New York State mental hospitals from 1955 to 1959 (Brill and Patton, 1959).

improvement was associated with a decrease in psychopathological symptoms.

There are numerous studies in which the association between the decrease in psychopathology and neuroleptic treatment—or increase in psychopathology with discontinuation of neuroleptic treatment—was shown. In the early 1960's in collaboration with the late Doctor Andre St. Jean, we were able to demonstrate that prolonged neuroleptic treatment has a therapeutic effect in chronically hospitalized schizophrenic patients. After a two-week drug-free interval, the seventy-one schizophrenic patients included in the study were administered one of three different phenothiazines, i.e. chlorpromazine (maximum 1500 mg/day) trifluoperazine (maximum 60 mg/day) or thioridazine (maximum 1500 mg/day) over a period of six months. Subsequently all patients were taken off medication for the next six months or until exacerbation of their illness. To our surprise, it was found that during the first three months of neuroleptic treatment, the patients, rather than improving, actually deteriorated (Fig. 17). During the next three months, however, there was a remarkable improvement which was seen in the decrease of mean total scores, from 8.3 to 4.1, on the Verdun Target Symptom Rating Scale (VTSRS) (Table VIII). This improvement was statistically significant at the 0.002 level of confidence. The patients maintained this improvement

TABLE VIII

VERDUN TARGET SYMPTOM RATING SCALE

---

1. Excitement
2. Suspiciousness
3. Hostility
4. Anxiety
5. Depression
6. Object relations
7. Hallucinations
8. Disturbance in thinking
9. Delusions
10. Memory disturbances
11. Impairment of consciousness
12. Impairment of expected social response
    Total

Scored from 0 to 3 (0, absent; 1, mild; 2, moderate; 3, severe).

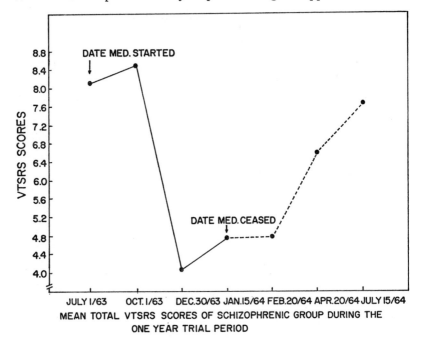

MEAN TOTAL VTSRS SCORES OF SCHIZOPHRENIC GROUP DURING THE
ONE YEAR TRIAL PERIOD

Figure 17. Mean total changes of VTSRS scores during the one-year experimental period.

for a month after medication ceased and then deteriorated almost to their pretrial level by the end of the six-month no-medication period. This deterioration also proved to be statistically significant ($p < 0.005$).

There is sufficient evidence to suggest that withdrawal of neuroleptic medication in chronically hospitalized schizophrenic patients leads to relapse in a considerable percentage of cases within a one-month- to a one-year period (Good, Sterling and Holtzman, 1958; Shawver *et al.*, 1959; Tuteur, Stiller and Glotzer, 1961; Morton, 1968). Relapse rate seems to be rather consistent, between 35 to 45 percent, by the end of the fourth month (Caffey *et al.*, 1964; Blackburn and Allen, 1961; Weiner and Feinberg, 1964; Rothstein, Zeltzerman and White 1962), while it varies from 40 percent (Prien *et al.*, 1968) to 75 percent (Olson and Petersen, 1960) by the end of the sixth month. In one of our recently completed studies with Doctor J. V. Ananth, only four (6.6 percent) of sixty chronically hospitalized schizophrenic patients could be maintained without medication without relapse over a one-year period.

Death Rate

Death rate of schizophrenics was consistently higher, especially in psychiatric hospitals, than in the general population in the prepsychopharmacological era. With the introduction of neuroleptic drugs, however, there seemed to be a further increase in sudden death, due to orthostatic hypotension, cardiac arrhythmias, cerebral seizures with regurgitation and asphyxia, in newly admitted cases. Thus there was the distinct possibility that the price for the increase in beneficial behavioral effects of neuroleptic drugs was an increase in death rate. For some time, there was no answer to the disturbing question of whether neuroleptic drug treatment increased mortality in the mental hospital. A rather long waiting period intervened until the first definitive paper on this rather serious problem was published (Turunen and Salminen, 1968). This report was based on 4625 patients, 2532 on neuroleptics and 2093 not on neuroleptics, hospitalized in the years from 1950 to 1964. During this time, there were 521 deaths in the total experimental population, 273 (i.e. 10.7 percent) in patients treated with neuroleptics and 243 (i.e. 11.6 percent) in those who were not on neuroleptics. The introduction of neuroleptics did not increase mortality, and if anything, it decreased mortality in hospitalized schizophrenic patients. The decrease in mortality rate, however, did not reach the accepted level of statistical significance.

In collaboration with Doctor Mohamed Amin, we became interested in studying changes in death rate at our own hospital (Douglas Hospital, Verdun), with special emphasis on the contingency of neuroleptic drugs. We have compared death rates for four five-year periods: 1930-1934 (base line), 1940-1944 (introduction of physical therapies), 1949-1953 (drug or therapeutic advances in general medicine) and 1956-1960 (introduction of neuroleptics) and found a significant decrease (and not increase) in mortality rates in the population under sixty-five years of age in the neuroleptic period, i.e. 1956-1960 (Fig. 18). Our findings were in full agreement with Turunen and Salminen's (1968) report. Furthermore, it was also noted that while the life expectancy of patients in mental hospitals in 1930-1934 was twelve years shorter than for Canadians on the whole, there was virtually no difference in life expectancy of the two populations in the

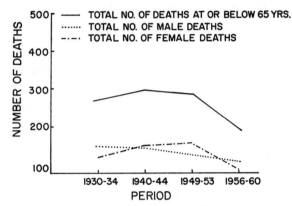

Figure 18. Total number of deaths in the population below 65 years of age at the Douglas Hospital in four time periods.

neuroleptic era. Finally, of the four periods, only in 1956-1960 was there no death due to exhaustion, and with the exception of the 1949-1953 period, only in the neuroleptic era was there any death ascribed (7 cases) to aspiration pneumonia.

In spite of the decreasing rate, there are still schizophrenic patients who die and whose death could be prevented by routinely employing EEG, EKG, and electrolyte (Na,K,Mg) determinations prior to and in the course of neuroleptic treatment (Laestma and Koenig, 1968). Cancro and Wilder (1970) suggests that death due to hypotensive reaction might be appreciably reduced by such simple means as repeated measurements for postural hypotension and sweating of the extremities during the first few days of psychopharmacological treatment.

Neuroleptics Versus Other Treatments

Simultaneous with the introduction of neuroleptics, there were radical changes in the organization of psychiatric care. It was suggested that these new administrative developments were rendered possible by the behavioral effects of the new drugs and that the resulting social changes in the hospitals have in turn helped to increase the efficacy of neuroleptic drugs. Nevertheless, others maintain that in some of the better-equipped hospitals where modern methods of treatment and adequately trained personnel in large enough numbers were available before the introduction of neuroleptics, the advantageous effects of these substances have been less impressive and that the therapeutic atmosphere of these institutions has not undergone much modification, either in respect to population dynamics or to the outcome of chronic psychoses.

Independent of the stand taken on the role of social changes in the new developments, there has been consensus that the introduction of neuroleptic drugs has eased the task of the nursing and medical staff (Chanoit *et al.*, 1970).

Social Therapies

Clinical studies could not substantiate the notion that the effect of neuroleptics is less apparent in better equipped hospitals, nor could they substantiate the notion that a better social milieu increases the effectiveness of neuroleptic drugs. In a study carried out by the National Institute of Mental Health Psychopharmacology Service Centre Collaborative Study Group at nine different locations, the effect of neuroleptics was no less apparent in the private hospitals than in state hospital settings (Scheflen, 1961).

It took considerably longer to clarify whether or not social therapies increase the efficacy of neuroleptic drugs. In favor of the view that social therapies increase the effectiveness of neuroleptics are Greenblatt and his collaborators (1965). In a 36-month study with 115 chronic schizophrenic patients they found that after six months, drug therapy was slighty more effective in association with social therapies (33 percent improvement) than when it was administered as the sole treatment (23 percent improvement). The same applied to the 36-month assessment. By that time, thirteen patients from the combined treatment group lived in the community, as compared to five patients from the group which received only neuroleptic treatment. The results of Greenblatt *et al.* (1965) were further substantiated by Borowski and Tolwinski's (1969) report, which showed that in paranoid schizophrenic patients, the combination of group therapy with chlorpromazine was superior to neuroleptic treatment alone. On the other hand, Evangelakis (1961), King (1963) and Gorham and Pokorny (1964) did not find a significant difference between treatment with neuroleptics alone and in combination with group therapy in schizophrenic patients.

The most comprehensive evaluation of milieu therapy, however, was carried out by May (1968) in a one-year comparative study of five different treatment regimes in 228 schizophrenic patients. He was able to demonstrate that for the "general run of schizophrenic patients" milieu therapy *alone* is both "expensive" and "relatively ineffective." In fact, of the five treatment regimes compared, milieu therapy alone was shown to be the least effective. These results gained further impetus with the report of Messier *et al.* (1969) which showed that the effectiveness of neuroleptic treatment in a group of chronic schizophrenic patients in an active therapeutic milieu was not significantly different than in the regular ward milieu of a local state hospital.

In view of the fact that of the five treatment regimes compared, milieu care alone is rather ineffective in the treatment of schizophrenic patients. May (1968) asserts that it is "fiscally unsound, penny-wise and pound foolish" to propose a budget that relies on milieu care primarily without adequate provision for appropriate neuroleptic treatment. To illustrate this, he pointed out that for the fiscal year of 1966, if the 3253 schizophrenic patients admitted to psychiatric hospitals were given a good level of milieu care alone, at an average per patient cost of 6230 dollars, it would have cost the state of California 20,270,000 dollars. By contrast, the cost of treating the same patients with neuroleptic drugs alone (which was found to be the most effective single form of specific treatment in his study) at an average per patient cost of 2960 dollars would have cost only 9,630,000 dollars; or treating the same patients with combined-individual psychotherapy plus neuroleptic drugs at an average per patient cost of 3640 dollars would have cost 11,840,000 dollars. Thus, in comparison with the cost of providing a good level of conservative milieu therapy, the net effect of using the most effective single treatment is a saving of 10,640,000 dollars per year, and the net effect of using the most effective combination is a saving of 8,430,000 dollars per year. This amount, May (1968) suggests, is roughly the same as the annual budget of two neuropsychiatric institutes in California.

Individual Psychotherapies

The fact that milieu therapy, the most expensive form of treatment, has the least therapeutic effect in schizophrenic patients called for a systematic reassessment of the value of the various contemporarily used treatment methods, i.e. psychotherapy, physical therapies and combined pharmacological treatments.

In regard to psychoanalysis, the most sophisticated of individual psychotherapies, it is well known that Freud himself saw little use for it in the "narcissistic neuroses"—his label for the schizophrenias. Since Freud, however, many psychotherapists have reported results, mainly anecdotal, supporting the effectiveness of psychotherapy in schizophrenic patients, but a recent comparative study at the Massachusetts Mental Health Center showed that psychotherapy conducted over a two-year period by experienced senior psychiatrists produced little change in chronic schizophrenic patients (while neuroleptic drugs did cause significant improvement on objective tests) (Greenblatt, 1968). Similarly, a five-year clinical follow-up study of schizophrenics treated by Rosen's "direct analysis" did not show significantly better results than a random control group or a designated control group (Bookhammer *et al.*, 1966).

In spite of the evidence that psychotherapy does little or nothing for schizophrenic patients, some psychotherapists still claim that pharmacotherapy interferes with psychotherapeutic progress, whatever this progress may be. Nevertheless, at least in one well-designed study, it was shown that actual facts are to the contrary.

The interaction between psychotherapy and neuroleptics was investigated by Grinspoon and Ewalt (1966) over a two-year period in chronic schizophrenic patients. At first, placebo was substituted for all neuroleptics in the total experimental population for a three-month period, and only afterwards was a neuroleptic (thioridazine) given to one half of the patients (while the other half were continued on the inactive preparation). As a result, it was found that patients given thioridazine did significantly better than patients treated with placebo, in spite of the fact that both groups received the same number of hours in intensive psychotherapy. Not only did pharmacotherapy not interfere with progress in psychotherapy but the administration of thioridazine made patients more "accessible" and also more receptive to communication with the psychotherapist (Grinspoon, Ewalt and Shader, 1968).

While there are indications that the administration of neuroleptic drugs may facilitate psychotherapy in schizophrenic patients, there is no evidence that psychotherapy would increase the effectiveness of pharmacological treatment. May and Tuma (1965), in their study with 100 first-admitted schizophrenic patients, found that patients treated with neuroleptic drugs with or without psychotherapy did significantly better than patients treated with milieu therapy alone. They could not find any significant difference between the two (with psychotherapy and without psychotherapy) drug-treated groups. Extension of this work to 228 patients did not improve the status of combined treatment. If anything, patients on the combination tended to stay longer in the hospital than patients who were given only drug treatment. This, together with the expense of psychiatric sessions, considerably escalated the cost of psychiatric services of patients on the combined treatment.

That psychotherapy might have a negative effect on neuroleptic treatment was contested by Karon and Vandenbos (1970). According to them, May's (1968) findings are skewed by the very fact that psychotherapy in May's (1968) study was conducted by "inexperienced therapists." Karon and Vandenbos (1970), in their own work, found that patients treated by experienced therapists with psychotherapy alone were hospitalized for a considerably shorter time than those treated by inexperienced therapists. Nevertheless, patients treated by inexperienced therapists utilizing neuroleptic medication in association with psychotherapy were hospitalized for even a shorter period than the patients of the experienced therapists (who were not using medication).

Physical Therapies

In contrast to the psychotherapies, there are definite indications that both physical therapies, i.e. insulin coma and electric shock, have a beneficial effect for schizophrenic patients.* While insulin-coma therapy was found to be equal in its therapeutic efficacy to

---

*It should be noted that Ackner and Oldham (1962) found no significant treatment difference in the improvement of a group of schizophrenic patients with insulin coma treatment over a control (barbiturate sedated) group; that Miller, Clancy and Cumming (1953) found no appreciable difference in the improvement of catatonics and a group of mixed psychotics with electroconvulsive treatment (ECT) over the control group of patients who received anesthesia alone; and that Letemendia and Harris (1967) in a double-blind placebo-controlled long-term clinical trial of chlorpromazine—in untreated chronic schizophrenic patients—following a methodologically sophisticated cross-over design, did not find statistically significant differences between the experimental and the control group.

neuroleptics in general and chlorpromazine and trifluoperazine in particular in numerous clinical studies (Baker, Game and Thorpe, 1958; Fink *et al.*, 1958; Markowe, Steinert and Heyworth-Davis, 1967; McNeill and Madgwick, 1961; Saarma, 1964) Kelly and Sargant (1965) gave conclusive evidence that insulin-coma treatment is less effective for schizophrenic patients than neuroleptic drugs.

They compared thirty-nine schizophrenic patients treated with insulin coma with eighty-four schizophrenics treated with various phenothiazines and found that of the insulin-treated group, 31 percent were in hospital (and 51 percent were rated as psychotic) at the two-year follow-up as compared with 7 percent in hospital (and 26 percent psychotic) in the phenothiazine-treated group. The average length of stay was also shorter in the phenothiazine-treated (6.7 weeks) group than in the insulin-coma-treated (10.7 weeks) group (Table IX).

TABLE IX

COMPARISON OF TREATMENT OUTCOME WITH INSULIN AND NEUROLEPTICS*

Treatment	In Hospital after 2 Years (% of Patients)	Psychotic after 2 Years (% of Patients)	Average Length of Stay in Hospital (in Weeks)
Insulin	31	51	10.7
Neuroleptics	7	26	6.7

*Kelly and Sargent, 1965.

The same applied to electroconvulsive treatment (ECT) as to insulin-coma therapy. While ECT was found to be equal to chlorpromazine, prochlorperazine, trifluoperazine or a combination of neuroleptics (Baker, Game and Thorpe, 1958; Rahman, 1968) or only slightly inferior to chlorpromazine (Langsley, Enterline and Hickerson, 1959; Riddell, 1963), May (1968) in a definitive study, established that ECT is less effective than neuroleptic drugs alone or neuroleptics in combination with psychotherapy in the treatment of schizophrenic patients (although it is more effective than milieu and/or individual psychotherapy) (Table X).

Finally, Smith *et al.* (1967) raised the possibility that ECT combined with antipsychotic drugs may be helpful; and Rahman (1968)

TABLE X

RELATIVE EFFECTIVENESS OF TREATMENT MODALITIES
IN SCHIZOPHRENICS

Neuroleptics > Neuroleptics > ECT > Individual psychotherapy > Milieu therapy + Psychotherapy

in his comparative study with 176 schizophrenic patients noted that
ECT combined with phenothiazines had a better therapeutic effect
than either ECT or any of the phenothiazines alone. This, however,
needs to be confirmed. In the meantime, ECT remains the treatment
of choice for those schizophrenic patients who develop toxic side
effects to drugs or for those who fail to respond to neuroleptics
alone or in combination with psychotherapy.

Pharmacological Treatments

Ever since it has been generally accepted that neuroleptics are the
primary form of treatment for schizophrenics, there has been an
increasing concern about the rather tight and frequent treatment
schedules, from three to four times a day, patients must follow in
their maintenance treatment. However, Brophy (1969) has shown
that in approximately 70 percent of chronic schizophrenic patients,
it is sufficient to administer neuroleptic medication just once a day,
and DiMascio and Shader (1969) brought to attention that chronic
schizophrenic patients can be maintained on intermittent drug treatment, starting with at least "drug-free weekends." Nevertheless, to
overcome the problem of tight and frequent treatment schedules,
an increasing number of long-acting neuroleptic preparations have
recently been developed. Among them, fluphenazine enanthate (maximum two weeks' duration) and decanoate (maximum ten weeks'
duration) have been introduced for general clinical use (Bankier,
Pettit and Bergen, 1968; Hsu *et al.*, 1967; Karkalas, 1968; Keskiner
et al., 1968; Kurland and Richardson, 1966; Miller and Daniel,
1967; Ravaris, Weaver and Brooks, 1967; Simpson *et al.*, 1965).
Both of these long-acting preparations seem to be equal in
their therapeutic efficacy to regularly administered neuroleptics, but
there are indications that they possibly produce a somewhat higher
incidence of adverse effects which call for discontinuation of treat-

ment, and a somewhat higher incidence of extrapyramidal signs which can only be controlled by the regular administration of anti-parkinsonian drugs (DeVerteuille *et al.*, 1970; Stewart and Lavallee, 1969; Whittier *et al.*, 1967). Because of these problems, the future of long-acting preparations depends on the actual percentage of psy-chiatric patients who abandon their medication.* Nevertheless, the fact remains that insofar as irregular or lapsed medication may have contributed to social maladjustment and readmission to hospital, long-acting neuroleptics could close an important gap (Roth, 1970).

Another popular topic is the question of drug combinations which would be particularly useful for therapeutic failures to one or another neuroleptic drug or for chronic patients who remained resistant be-yond a certain point to the therapeutic effects of drugs, i.e. failed to respond sufficiently to be discharged. Of the numerous combina-tions tried, including anxiolytic sedatives with neuroleptics, stimu-lants with neuroleptics, antidepressants with neuroleptics, and neuro-leptics with neuroleptics (Ban, 1969a; Casey *et al.*, 1961; Cole and Davis, 1969; Michaux, Kurland and Agallianos, 1966), only the combination of perphenazine with amitriptyline (neuroleptic with antidepressant) and the combination of chlorpromazine with triflu-operazine (neuroleptic with neuroleptic) seemed to be of clinical significance (Freeman, 1967; Hanlon *et al.*, 1964; Nemeth and Petro-wich, 1967; Swanson, Smith and Perez, 1967). Nevertheless, neither of these combinations was found to be superior in therapeutic effi-cacy to the administration of either drug alone (Gardos, Rapkin and DiMascio, 1968; Hollister *et al.*, 1963; Oltman and Friedman, 1966). On the other hand, the increase of daily chlorpromazine dos-age to 2000 mg/day was shown to be significantly more effective than routine treatment, at least in patients under forty years of age and with less than ten years of hospitalization (Prien and Cole, 1968).

SPECIFIC EFFECTS

While describing the reduction of both short- and long-term hos-pital stays in the psychopharmacological era, Kelly and Sargant (1965) brought to attention that the percentage of "symptom-free"

*Hare and Wilcox (1967) found that 19 percent of inpatients and 37 percent of outpatients fail in taking medication regularly, and McClelland and Cowan (1970) reported that 8 percent of patients report inaccurately the amount of medication taken.

schizophrenic patients has not been increased by the introduction of neuroleptic drugs and that the improvements have been confined to a shift from the prevalence of "psychotic" to the prevalence of "residual" symptoms. Prior to this, a similar notion was expressed by Sargant and Slater (1963), who asserted that neuroleptic drugs halt the schizophrenic process and lessen the chance of chronic illness as well as personality deterioration, but they do not cure the schizophrenic patient. Malitz (1964) also suggested that neuroleptic drugs reduce quantitatively the overt manifestations of the schizophrenic process without eliminating or correcting it.

Changes in Patients

Syndromes

Fouks *et al.* (1966) have pointed out that the distinction between acute and chronic psychoses often disappears with modern pharmacotherapy which tends to inhibit the evolution of schizophrenic symptoms and halt the natural course toward chronicity. This dedifferentiation of psychotic manifestations is probably one of the reasons that first-admitted schizophrenics are diagnosed, almost exclusively, as paranoid and undifferentiated since the introduction of neuroleptic drugs (Hogarty and Gross, 1966). Accordingly Stone *et al.* (1968) suggest that there are no real examples of simple schizophrenia.

Another observation that has been shared by all who have treated schizophrenics with neuroleptic drugs is the modification of chronic and terminal stages of progressive schizophrenia (Lehmann, 1969a). This is, in part, related to the interference by psychopharmacological means with the progress of the disease (Fouks *et al.*, 1966) and related also to the action of prolonged drug treatment which tends to produce a pattern of retarded, abulic behavior—a reduction of energy potential—which is due to a suppression of productive symptoms (Huber, 1964). Some considered the marked decrease in all psychotic symptoms from first admission to rehospitalization (Morgan, Porzio and Hedlund, 1968) as the result of this "retarded, abulic behavior." While before neuroleptics the schizophrenic process was characterized by a gradual loss of active symptoms and the late appearance of a typical defect syndrome, in the psychopharmacological era it is characterized by abrupt abolishment of acute symptoms and interference, possibly even indefinite postponement of the typical defect syndrome.

In a recent publication, Vartanian (1968) discussed the "therapeutic pathomorphosis" of "terminal schizophrenia" and gave an account of a release of productive symptoms after discontinuation of long-term drug therapy in thirty-five patients who were in advanced stages of schizophrenia. While prior to treatment it had been assumed that productive symptoms in these patients were irreversibly extinguished, Vartanian (1968) recognized that they had only been masked by the effects of neuroleptic drugs.

Another evidence that the nosological groups of acute and chronic schizophrenia have not been abolished by neuroleptics was given by Astrup (1962). In his monograph *Schizophrenia Conditional Reflex Studies,* he was able to classify acute schizophrenic patients according to Schneider (1942) and chronic schizophrenic patients according to Leonhard's (1936) criteria and describe the differential conditional reflex profiles of these clinical categories (Tables XI and XII). The single fact that it was possible to classify patients into all of Schneider's and Leonhard's groups indicates that in spite of all the blurring effect of neuroleptics, the mask created in the psychopharmacological era, all of the classes of schizophrenia still exist.

There is, however, at least one definite area in which the nosological groups of today differ from the nosological groups described sixty years ago. In Kraepelin's (1910) time, paranoid schizophrenics carried the worst prognosis and catatonics the best, the hebephrenics being inbetween. On the other hand, both Achté (1961) and Holmboe and Astrup (1957) found that today hebephrenic patients have the worst prognosis and catatonics the best. But it seems to be that this prognostic shift had already started prior to the introduction of neuroleptic drugs.

Symptoms

To see whether schizophrenic symptoms had changed over an interval of a century, including the beginning of the psychopharmacological era, Klaf and Hamilton (1961) compared the records of patients admitted to the Bethlehem Hospital during 1853 to 1862 and 1950 to 1960. They found that the proportion of acutely disturbed

TABLE XI

NUMBER OF ACUTE AND SUBACUTE SCHIZOPHRENIC PATIENTS INCLUDED IN ASTRUP'S (1962) SYSTEMATIC CONDITIONING STUDY*

Group	Number of Patients
1. Hebephrenic and hebephrenic paranoid psychoses	40
2. Catatonic and mixed catatonic psychoses	44
3. Paranoid psychoses dominated by projection symptoms	51
4. Paranoid psychoses with systematized delusions	43
Total	178

*Patients were grouped according to Carl Schneider's (1942) classification.

TABLE XII

NUMBER OF CHRONIC SCHIZOPHRENIC PATIENTS INCLUDED IN ASTRUP'S SYSTEMATIC CONDITIONING STUDY*

Subgroups	Hebephrenia (No. of Pts.)	Systematic Catatonia (No. of Pts.)	Systematic Paraphrenia (No. of Pts.)
1. Autistic	7		
2. Eccentric	17		
3. Shallow	12		
4. Silly	14		
5. Periodic		16	
6. Parakinetic		14	
7. Speech-prompt		12	
8. Proskinetic		14	
9. Speech-inactive		18	
10. Negativistic		10	
11. Manneristic		17	
12. Affect-laden			22
13. Schizophasia			15
14. Phonemic			19
15. Hypochondriacal			16
16. Expansive and confabulatory			13
17. Fantastic			16
18. Incoherent			15

*Patients were grouped according to Leonhard's (1936) classification.

patients, on admission, was considerably higher in the earlier (60 percent) than in the later (8 percent) group; and that religious preoccupation was three times as frequent in the 1850's than in the 1950's, while sexual preoccupation was twice as frequent in the 1950's than in the 1850's. Similarly to Lucas, Sainsbury and Collins (1962), who have shown that the content of schizophrenic delusions varied with social background—for example, religious preoccupation was common in single persons, while grandiose ideas were common in patients of a higher social status—Klaf and Hamilton (1961) concluded that the changes in the content of schizophrenic delusions and hallucinations were determined by cultural factors and were independent from the introduction of neuroleptics. They made no attempt, however, to decide whether the decrease in acutely disturbed patients on admission in the later group was related to the introduction of neuroleptic drugs or to the social changes which have taken place between the 1850's and the 1950's.

An entirely different aspect of changes which have occurred during the last 100 years in psychopathological symptoms was presented by Ödegard (1967). He gave a descriptive account of the typical deteriorated schizophrenic patient of Kraepelin's time who stood around in the wards without any orderly activity, was incontinent, passive and cataleptic, had to be fed, dressed and washed and who mumbled incomprehensibly, and pointed out that only a very few of these classical patients are still around, as leftovers from the prepsychopharmacological era (or even from the period before the somatic therapies were introduced). Because of the scarcity of these patients, it is difficult to find cases with the classical textbook symptoms, as, for example, mutism, negativism, incoherence, catalepsy, or other catatonic features, such as flexibilitas cerea, stereotypes, regressive incontinence and aggressive-impulsive behavior. In spite of this, Ödegard (1967) asserts that on the whole, the change over the years in the schizophrenic defect picture is of a quantitative nature, i.e. the defect is still the same but by losing its "physiogenic" character, has changed in degree. The instability of therapeutic results and the strong tendency towards psychotic relapse are warning signals, however, that schizophrenia is more than a psychogenic reaction on the surface. Nevertheless, the fact remains that the transformation of schizophrenic defect states began well before the psychopharmacological era, and even if the introduction of neuroleptics greatly contributed to the changes, the new picture cannot be attributed entirely to the therapeutic effects of new drugs.

In contrast to Ödegard (1967), who emphasized the importance of changes in social attitudes, Snezhnevski (1965) asserts that the introduction of psychopharmacological agents has an exclusive role in the transformation of psychopathological symptoms in schizophrenic patients. According to him, there is sufficient clinical evidence to repudiate that neuroleptics are merely symptomatic drugs and to demonstrate that they are antipathogenic agents which, by acting on symptoms, affect the links in the "pathogenetic chain" of the pathological process in schizophrenia. Accordingly, Snezhnevski (1965) suggests that under the influence of neuroleptics, (a) the "development stereotype" of schizophrenia has changed and the schizophrenic process, i.e. recurrent episodes with progressive deterioration, has been replaced by schizophrenic shifts, i.e. recurrent episodes with partial recovery, (b) that the "disease stereotype" of schizophrenia has changed and the prevailing picture of "systematized delusions and hallucinations" has been replaced by a "depressive-paranoid" disorder, and (c) that the transformation of minor, i.e. more homogenous, clinical manifestations, into major, i.e. more complex, clinical syndromes has stopped or even reversed. Furthermore, he asserts that all pathological productive symptoms, e.g. psychic automatisms, paraphrenic delusions and schizophasia, of schizophrenia can be *controlled* by persistent and prolonged neuroleptic treatment, and all pathological deficit signs, e.g. mental defects and withdrawal, can be *corrected* to a certain degree. As a result of this, Snezhnevski (1965) maintains that the manifestations of schizophrenic defect states have changed and are characterized by signs of "ontogenetic regression" in general and by signs of "psychic infantilism and juvenilism" in particular. Nevertheless, the fact remains that at least some of these changes, e.g. increase in the occurrence of depressions and/or paranoid manifestations, began well before the psychopharmacological era.

The idea that schizophrenic psychopathological symptoms and not only schizophrenic defect states are the result of ontogenetic regression is not new, and it had already been entertained prior to the psychopharmacological era. Nyirö (1958) formulated a most comprehensive theory to explain the various psychopathological symptoms of schizophrenia as "regressive" and "dissociative" manifestations. He put forward a "structural view" which was based on the three phases of the reflex mechanism and pointed out the similarity of the proposed structure to three pyramids, the cognitive, the relational and the adaptive (Fig. 19). He suggested that differential inhibition and retarded (or delayed) inhibition play prominent roles in the formation of the pyramids and in the formation of interpyramidal connections respectively. Accordingly, Nyirö (1958) maintains that schizophrenic episodes are characterized by interpyramidal "dissociations"; the thrusts, by progressive "regression" from a higher to a lower pyramidal level; and schizophrenic defect states, by fixation on a low-regressed pyramidal level. There are indications that the severity of regression is alleviated by neuroleptic drugs. Systematic observations of schizophrenic patients in the neuroleptic era, applying this frame of reference, revealed that most of the clinically employed neuroleptic preparations interfered with perceptual disorders and thought disorders in general and also with the pathological release of uncoordinated motor movements and emotional-instinctual stereotypes. Withdrawal of the same medications resulted in the recurrence of hallucinations, delusions and blocking as well as the recurrence of excitement, agitation, and a variety of catatonic manifestations. It was also noted that while sensory hallucinations are interfered with by neuroleptics, coenestopathies are not (Nyirö, 1958; Ekdawi, 1966; Hoehn-Saric and Gross, 1968; Gottschalk *et al.*, 1970). Since some of these changes had already begun prior to the psychopharmacological era, the question remains as to which of these changes can be attributed to the introduction of neuroleptic drugs.

While it is difficult to decide with certainty which of the changes in psychopathological symptoms are directly related to the introduction of neuroleptic drugs, there are indications of differences in psychopathological symptom profiles, in the prepsychopharmacological and psychopharmacological era. Among the differences most prevalent is the decrease of catatonic and the increase of paranoid syndromes in the psychopharmacological era; however, this shift in symptomatology may well have been the result of time-related and cultural factors, rather than due to the effects of neuroleptics. The

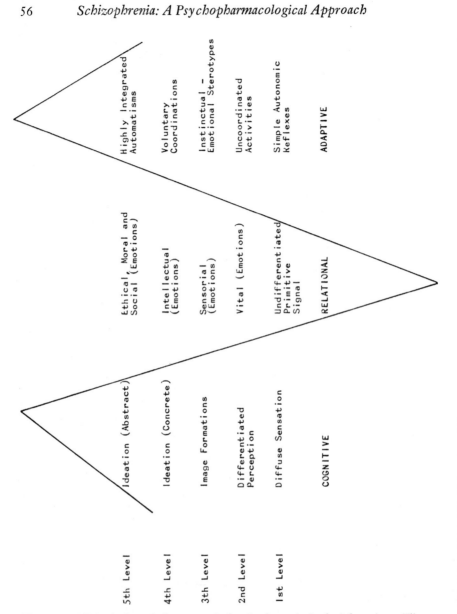

Figure 19. Nyirö's (1958) "structural view" of psychological functions. The three structures, cognitive, relational and adaptive, resemble three pyramids with the apex of the one in the middle turned downwards.

same applies to depressions which seem to occur more frequently in schizophrenics today than before the introduction of neuroleptic drugs (Achté, 1961; Battegay and Gehring, 1968; Bohacek, 1965; Bowers and Astrachan, 1967; Lehmann, 1969a, b; Steinberg, Green and Durell, 1967; Varga, 1966).

The most definitive study to date in the differentiation of the therapeutic effects of neuroleptics and nonspecific factors, e.g. placebo in schizophrenic patients, was reported by Goldberg, Klerman and Cole (1965). They were able to demonstrate that there is a group of psychiatric symptoms in schizophrenics, consisting of irritability, slow speech and movements, hebephrenic symptoms, self-care and indifference to environment, in which there is no improvement except on drug treatment. Goldberg, Klerman and Cole (1965) also suggested that these symptoms are related to Bleuler's (1911) fundamental symptoms in schizophrenia, i.e. loosening of association, ambivalence and inappropriateness of affect, and autism, in contradistinction to the placebo-prone symptoms such as auditory and nonauditory hallucinations, memory deficit and feelings of unreality, which are closely related to Bleuler's (1911) accessory symptoms, i.e. hallucinations, delusions and catatonic symptoms. On the basis of these findings, they suggested that the frequently held view that phenothiazine effects are only symptomatic and that they "dampen" only the accessory or manifest symptoms without having an effect on the fundamental disease process is probably wrong and needs to be reevaluated (Table XIII). This corresponds with Snezhnevski's thesis that neuroleptics are more than symptomatic agents for schizophrenic patients. Nevertheless, the relationship between Goldberg, Klerman and Cole's (1965) drug-dependent and Bleuler's (1911) fundamental symptoms is far from being established and even if it will be supported by further evidence, the selective action of neuroleptics on these symptoms will have to be confirmed.

SOCIAL EFFECTS

Schizophrenics in the Community

Personality-Specific Changes

One of the definite characteristics of the psychopharmacological era is the decreasing percentage of schizophrenics in psychiatric hos-

TABLE XIII

DRUG- (EXCLUSIVELY) AND PLACEBO-RESPONSIVE PSYCHOPATHO-
LOGICAL SYMPTOMS AND THEIR RELATIONSHIP TO BLEULER'S (1911)
FUNDAMENTAL AND ACCESSORY SYMPTOMS*

| Drug Responsive (Only) | *Symptoms* | | |
	Placebo Responsive	Fundamental (Bleuler)	Accessory (Bleuler)
Irritability	Auditory halluci- nations	Loosening of association	Hallucinations
Slow speech and movement	Nonauditory hallu- cinations	Ambivalence and inappropriateness of effect	Delusions
Hebephrenic symptoms	Memory defect	Autism	Catatonic symptoms
Self-care	Feeling of uncer- tainty		
Indifference to environment			

*In Goldberg, Klerman and Cole's (1965) study.

pitals and the increasing percentage of schizophrenics in the community. The majority of these patients are far from being cured, but they are, at least while they are taking their neuroleptic medication, sufficiently free of psychopathological manifestations to be able to cope, in most cases with some assistance, with the external world. There is a great variation in the personality of schizophrenic patients who live in the community which ranges from a very slight alteration in the individual, due to a reduction in understandability, to an almost complete fragmentation of personality. It is rather difficult to identify a common feature in the personality of all patients. If anything, there seems to be a kind of inability to recognize reality as reality and take it properly into account. In terms of the effect on the observer, most of these patients in the community have something baffling about them, which baffles understanding in a peculiar way; there is something queer, cold, inaccessible, rigid and petrified there, even when they are quite sensible and eager to talk about their problems. If there were a single uniform world formation in schizophrenics, one could hope that schizophrenics would understand at least each other. But this is not the case, and, if anything, a healthy person understands them better (Jaspers, 1962). There is little change in this respect in the psychopharmacological era. Furthermore, like in the prepsychopharmacological era, schizophrenics still do not talk freely about all the details of their illness and even if they do, it is usually accompanied by inappropriate excitement.

There is an excellent sketch by Ödegard (1967) on discharged, but not cured, patients. According to him, they are easily recognizable in the community by their stiffness and lack of spontaneity. They perform routine work with considerable skill, but because of a certain lack of initiative and decrease in speed, even if they find employment, they are usually rather soon dismissed. They are tactless, inconsiderate, indifferent, irritable at home, and all their old hobbies are gone while no new hobbies or interests have been developed. The development of these personality changes could not be prevented by neuroleptics alone. Nor is there evidence that they could be prevented by any other form of treatment.

Drug-Specific Changes

Superimposed on the personality changes are the possible adverse effects of neuroleptic treatment which may affect any organ or organ system, causing mild discomfort or infrequently severe pathological changes. Neuroleptic-induced extrapyramidal manifestations, i.e. akinesia, akathisia, tremor, rigidity, dystonia and parkinsonism, are very frequent, while neuroleptic-induced pyramidal damage or disturbing paresthesias are extremely rare. Cerebral seizures occur only in some predisposed cases (Ban, 1969a; Bishop, Gallant and Sykes, 1965; Pryce and Edwards, 1966; Roxburgh, 1970; Sheppard and Merlis, 1967); and orthostatic hypotension occurs, if at all, during the first few days of treatment. While autonomic and endocrine reactions (e.g. nasal congestion, dry mouth, blurred vision, amenorrhea, galactorrhea, swollen breasts) are rather frequent, agranulocytosis, obstructive jaundice, quinidine-like effects on the ECG and pigmentary retinopathy are rather rare (Bloom, Davis and Wecht, 1965; Fieve, Blumenthal and Little, 1966; Hagopian, Stratton and Busiek, 1966; Hollister and Hall, 1966; Lapierre *et al.*, 1969; Mandel and Gross, 1968; McKinney and Kane, 1967). A high percentage of patients complain of constipation and in spite of all the warnings, photosensitivity reactions (sunburn) and heat strokes still occur (Korenyi, 1969; Zelman and Guillan, 1970). There are indications that neuroleptics may precipitate latent diabetes mellitus (and also bronchial asthma) (Korenyi and Lowenstein, 1968; Thonnard-Neumann, 1968; Dynes, 1969). While the patient is in hospital, these adverse effects are discomforting; in the community they are also interfering with the social activities of schizophrenic patients.

Drug-Patient Interaction

The psychotropic properties of neuroleptics cannot be reduced to a single chemical, neurophysiological or psychophysiological concomitant of drug action. On the neurochemical level, there is central adrenergic blocking and stabilization of the membranes of the synaptic clefts, which by preventing the access of norepinephrine to the NE receptors, decreases neural transmission. On the neurophysiological level, there is stimulation of the amygdaloid nucleus (limbic system), depression of the hypothalamus and depression of the reticular activating system (or rather interference with the impulses of the afferent pathways to the brain-stem reticular formation). While the neurochemical action of these drugs on brain amines is usually considered to be related to their therapeutic action on "psychotic" manifestations, their neurophysiological effect on the three major integrating systems in the brain is usually considered to be responsible for their effect in diminishing the emotional response to stimuli from both the "external and the internal world" (Hollister, 1970a, b). Some consider that the problem in arousing schizophrenic patients in the mornings and the difficulty in getting them out of bed is related to the neurophysiological sites of action, while others maintain that the problem of arousal in the mornings had already been present prior to the introduction of neuroleptics.

On the psychophysiological level, while neuroleptics interfere with conditional reflex behavior, they leave unconditional reflex behavior virtually unaffected. Furthermore, while they have a marked inhibitory effect on the motor components of the conditional withdrawal reflex (Courvoisier, 1956), they affect the concomitant autonomic components of the same reflex to a much lesser extent (Tedeschi, Tedeschi and Fellows, 1961). This, at least in part, explains the significant reduction of pathological behavioral responses to conditional cues (stimuli) after the introduction of neuroleptic drugs. It also explains why schizophrenics do not respond to conditional cues of everyday life. That schizophrenics stand out in any community they are in is not new. Foucault (1965) described the situation which arose when, in eighteenth-century France, criminals, schizophrenics and the indigent were all locked up together—the schizophrenics quickly became highly visible because they could not conform to the daily prison life. The problem in conforming to any social situation in the prepsychopharmacological era was primarily due to pathological behavioral responses to a variety of the unidentified conditional cues, while in the psychopharmacological era, it has been identified more as a deficit phenomenon, i.e not responding at all or at least not in an accepted manner to the cues of everyday life. For example, a young schizophrenic man of high intelligence gave an account of how difficult it was for him to respond to people and his environment in the manner in which he responded prior to his illness and as he consciously knew that he was expected to respond. He complained that dealing with people exhausted him, completely wore him out, to the extent that he sometimes wished to be back in the hospital. The only thing which helped him to cope with this situation was the possibility of getting away, "doing nothing but walk." He did this for 30 to 38 percent of his time, well within the range of 21 to 43 percent walking time reported in long-stay schizophrenic inpatients (Wing, 1967). He had had sexual preoccupations since his adolescence, which prior to his illness were primarily focused on a premature ejaculation pattern. With neuroleptics, the situation reversed and went to the other extreme. More important, he observed that no olfactory, visual or tactile—him touching her—stimuli could elicit in him an erection. Erection was only obtained by persistent manual stimulation—her touching him—and ejaculation was achieved by a certain quantity of friction without any of the psychological emotional concomitants of orgasm. While he was preoccupied with sex and was able to perform and satisfy, he was not able to achieve any pleasure or satisfaction himself. Naturally, this loss of feeling of pleasure (anhedonia) in schizophrenics is not new. A long time before the psychopharmacological era, Hölderlin, who experienced this himself (Jaspers, 1962), expressed it by simple and moving words: "July and June and May / have gone so far away. / I have no more to give. / I do not want to live." (Free translation by H. E. Lehmann.)

In contrast to Kraepelin's (1896) and Bleuler's (1911) time, the typical schizophrenic today spends most of his lifetime outside the hospital in the community. They are rather "expensive" for the community they live in. In Walter and McCourt's (1965) study, for example, less than half of the patients (47 percent) were employed at any time after their discharge from hospital; and even if they obtained employment, only a small percentage, one fifth of the entire population, worked at a regular full-time job throughout the six-month follow-up period. More important, however, is that while in the community, they contaminate the genetic pool by their increase in fertile marriages (Erlenmeyer-Kimling *et al.*, 1969) and also contaminate the environment by their peculiar patterns of behavior. Where all this will lead nobody knows.

New Ideologies

Schizophrenia is a common disease. Its incidence per year is about 0.15 percent, its prevalence 0.3 percent and the lifetime probability for any individual to suffer a schizophrenic breakdown about 1 to 2 percent. There are approximately 600,000 schizophrenics in the United States (70,000 in Canada) and more than 200,000 Americans (20,000 Canadians) are presently hospitalized with one or another form of schizophrenia (Lehmann, 1969b; Mosher, 1969). There has been no change in these figures in the psychopharmacological era. There is sufficient evidence that at least certain productive psychopathological symptoms can be controlled by drugs, while first-year relapse rate can be cut from 40 to 75 to 5 to 15 percent with maintenance treatment. Neuroleptics, together with the improvement of milieu in psychiatric hospitals, have considerably transformed the prevailing manifestations of the disease, while the changes in social attitude, together with neuroleptic treatment, have produced an absolute and relative increase in schizophrenic patient population in the community. The reflection of these changes in consciousness led to new ideologies of mental illness in general and schizophrenia in particular. Among the first ideologists was Szasz (1961), himself a professor of psychiatry, who argued that psychiatry, which deals with "problems in living," is inappropriately subsumed under medicine and that behavior that we call "sick," e.g. schizophrenic behavior, is not physiologically determined.

While Szasz (1961) considered mental illness a myth, Scheff (1970), a professor of sociology, asserts that mental illness is nothing but a label for a wide "residual" category of social offenders. According to him, every society provides its members with a set of *explicit* norms (understandings governing conduct), and offenses against these norms have conventional names, e.g. theft, perversion. Beyond the explicit norms and their "conventional" offenses, every society has a countless number of unnamed understandings, and offenses against these unnamed residual understandings are usually lumped together in a residual category. He considers mental illness as the residual category in contemporary society and conceives the symptoms of mental illness in general and schizophrenia in particular as offenses (violations) against implicit social understandings. Scheff (1970) interprets the disordered speech and communication of schizophrenics as offenses against culturally prescribed roles of language and expression. Schizophrenic withdrawal, in his interpretation, assumes a "cultural standard, concerning the degree of involvement and the amount of distance between the individual and those around him." Furthermore, Scheff (1970) suggests that the societal reaction against these offenses of implicit social understandings is denial (i.e. ignoring or rationalizing) or labeling. If labeling occurs, the offender is labeled as mentally ill and is launched on a career of chronic punishment.

Similar views were expressed by Laing (1967), himself a psychoanalyst, who defined schizophrenia as a label which some people pin on other people under certain social circumstances. He believes that schizophrenia is not an illness but "a social fact and a political event." The goal of labeling schizophrenics is to maintain the status quo by "treating as medical patients certain individuals who, assumedly because of the strength of their inner perceptions and experiences, are exceptionally eloquent social critics" (Siegler, Osmond and Mann, 1969). Besides accepting schizophrenics as rebels, Laing (1967) also offers them a status above normal people. In his essay on "Politics of Experience," he redefines schizophrenia and suggests that it is a "natural way of healing our own appalling state of alienation called normality." Accordingly, schizophrenia is not an illness but a "voyage of inner exploration" on which "often through quite ordinary people," now called schizophrenics, "the light begins to break through the cracks in our all-too-closed minds."

The view that schizophrenia is not so much a breakdown as a breakthrough is shared by Dabrowski (1964, 1967), also a psychiatrist. He called it "positive disintegration" and considered it as a natural reaction to stress, which replaces usual problem-solving techniques in severe life crises. Furthermore, Silverman (1970), a psychologist, asserts that neuroleptics, by reducing the clarity of ordinary experience, interfere with schizophrenia's problem-solving process.

A common characteristic of these ideologies is that they adopt a view in opposition to the medical model. Nevertheless, they reflect a period in which the majority of schizophrenic patients can and are living outside of hospitals, a period in which schizophrenia is losing its "physiogenic" character and in which the progress of the schizophrenic process can be prevented and psychopathological symptoms alleviated. Social-environmental changes were instrumental in this evolution of events, but without neuroleptics, the present state of affairs could not have been reached. Still, the problem is that even with neuroleptics, very little has been achieved. To exaggerate the little we have achieved and claim that schizophrenia now does not exist is more than ideology—it is a falsehood which is corrected in the context of an alleged "truth" represented by an alleged "objective social interest." Nevertheless, if this falsehood would ever prevail, it would withhold progress towards an understanding of schizophrenia and the schizophrenic patient and could lead to a situation which is contrary to any social interest.

Chapter 4

SCHIZOPHRENIAS

ORGANIZATION OF PSYCHIATRIC SERVICES

W<small>HILE</small> no one would doubt that the introduction of chlorpromazine and subsequently of other neuroleptic drugs brought about important changes by effectively controlling certain symptoms of schizophrenia, there is little evidence of any fundamental breakthrough in our understanding of schizophrenia in the psychopharmacological era. On the other hand, within approximately ten years, it became generally accepted that by using neuroleptics, the majority of schizophrenic patients could be treated without hospitalization. To render psychiatric services accessible in the community, the organization of a new type of administrative mechanism began.

As a result of these "community organizations," the practice of psychiatry is expected to change. The actual demand by the communities to treat their most severely sick members, together with a shortage of professional personnel, will lead psychiatrists to change priorities not only among various forms of treatment but also among various types of patients who need to be first attended. This transformation cannot take place without a thorough transformation of psychiatric education.

Nevertheless, therapy-resistant cases will still remain and to prevent the reoccurrence of the old situation, i.e. accumulation of a large number of chronic patients, they will have to be transferred to highly specialized institutions of adequate size to provide economically for both optimal care and research (Ban, 1971).

METHODOLOGICAL PROBLEMS

A rather large number of neuroleptic drugs were synthesized and clinically introduced subsequent to chlorpromazine. These new drugs represented a variety of chemical structures and distinct biochemical,

65

neurophysiological and pharmacological effects. Nevertheless, the differences in the efficacy or in the differential therapeutic activity of these drugs remained hidden by the application of contemporary methods, to the extent that differential prescription of neuroleptics was usually based on their differential adverse, and not on their differential therapeutic, effects.

As psychopharmacology progressed, psychiatric and consequently clinical psychopharmacological work became increasingly disciplined by inductive logic which led to the utilization of the statistical method for the analysis of controlled clinical studies with neuroleptics in order to draw general conclusions on the basis of limited experimental samples. Needless to say, the requirements of a controlled experiment in which one variable, altered by the experimenter, is measured against a fixed background are far from being fulfilled in clinical psychopharmacological experimentation. Because of this, and probably even more so because of the absence of criteria for selecting truly homogeneous populations, all psychopharmacological studies with neuroleptics, even those conducted under the best possible conditions, fail to give a valid estimation of experimental error and to provide a genuine baseline for comparing the efficacy of the investigational substance with no treatment, a placebo, or a standard comparison drug. Thus, inductive logic, i.e. the rigid adherence to the scientific-statistical method, at this stage of development may well lead psychopharmacology into a deadlock.

Independent of this, the statistical method has its own shortcomings which might be responsible for the blurring of differential effects of neuroleptics. Among these are the type-I or alpha error, i.e. the finding of statistically significant difference when no difference actually exists, or the type-II or beta error, i.e. not finding statistically significant difference when an actual difference does exist. Thus, for example, on the basis of empirical analysis it was suggested that approximately 40 to 50 schizophrenic patients are required for each treatment group in a controlled double-blind study with neuroleptics in which the Brief Psychiatric Rating Scale is employed (Overall and Gorham, 1962; and Overall and Hollister, 1967). It is argued that below this sample size, the chance of beta error is so high that it would put the validity of the findings into question. Since it is impossible to clinically pursue at any acceptable level of thoroughness more than fifteen to thirty schizophrenic patients in any single drug trial, this sample size requirement for a controlled clinical study cannot be fulfilled within the frame of reference of the traditional approach.

Some of the more general pitfalls of the statistical method were perhaps best expressed by Huntsman (1949) who said that "the prestige of mathematics is so great that many persons forget that even in mathematical hands, probability, chance and random mean ignorance. They come to think that in the alembic of mathematics, chance in some way becomes certainty. They take great care to select random samples without realizing that insofar as a sample has been random, they don't know how it was selected." A more severe criticism was launched recently in *Lancet* by Wiener (1962). He pointed out that many clinical investigators, "because they are unduly sensitive or insecure regarding their lack of mathematics training and knowledge, habitually hand over all their data to biometricians for analysis in order that their papers may include the appropriate chi-square tests, standard errors and so on. In that way they have come to depend more and more on mathematicians who have no knowledge or understanding of the subject to interpret their findings, instead of relying on their own experience and common sense." In essence, Wiener (1962) attempts to remind the clinical investigator that mathematics is a poor substitute for accurate observations, reliable experimentation and common sense.

The dissatisfaction with the presently employed clinical methodology was reflected in a recent Psychopharmacological Attitude Poll (Lehmann, 1968). It was found that about 50 percent of the leading psychopharmacologists in North America would not consider the negative findings of a clinical drug trial performed under ideal experimental conditions as definitive if these negative findings were contradicted by two competent clinicians on the basis of their personal, uncontrolled experience. About 15 percent of psychopharmacologists would use the drug and thus indicate that they trust the experience of two clinicians more than the results of one controlled evaluation. Less than 10 percent of the total sample of psychopharmacologists would be sufficiently convinced by the outcome of the controlled experiment to discard the favorable impressions of the two clinicians entirely. Thus, the results of this inquiry demonstrate that the negative findings of a controlled clinical evaluation do not carry as much weight as positive findings of an uncontrolled nature if they are reported by competent clinicians. All of this clearly shows that clinical methodology has serious problems.

Allusions are frequently made that it is adherence to the "medical model" rather than to the scientific-statistical method that is responsible to the impasse in clinical psychopharmacology and clinical psychiatry. But psychiatry has actually never operated strictly within the medical model; its language was derived from philosophy which substantially determined its thinking and course of development. By now, there is abundant evidence that psychoactive drugs don't speak or share the language of psychiatry and that future progress in this discipline will depend greatly on the speed with which we develop a common language which will bridge the gap between psychiatry and the action of psychoactive drugs.

NEW APPROACHES

Pragmatic Considerations

It is often seen in schizophrenia research that the independent variable in the research design, e.g. the hypothetical cause of schizophrenia, is measured with considerable attention to reliability, validity and precision, yet the measurement of the dependent variable, the diagnosis of schizophrenia, is almost ignored. Naturally, the precision of the measurement is virtually nil, since it represents at best an ordinal scale or, much more likely, a nominal scale (Scheff, 1970).

The precision in the measurement of the dependent variable, i.e. diagnostic classification in schizophrenia, gains particular impetus if one considers that what is called schizophrenia is likely to be a group of diseases. There is no single physiological or biochemical hypothesis to date which applies to all the various forms of schizophrenias. On the contrary, there is increasing evidence that the clinical varieties are varied, like the physiological and biochemical changes. It is indeed likely that there are numerous schizophrenias, one of which responds best to phenothiazines, i.e. to chemicals which reduce arousal reaction (related to brain-stem reticular formation functioning), block adrenergic intrareticular mechanisms and decrease the cortical release of acetylcholine. Another may respond best to neuroleptic *Rauwolfia* alkaloids which, unlike the phenothiazines, exert a stimulating effect on the mesencephalic alerting system, facilitating the transmission of impulses in these areas (Rinaldi and Himwich, 1955), release various amines from their cellular storage sites and decrease brain 5-hydroxy-tryptamin (5-HT), norepinephrine and γ-aminobutyric acid (GABA) levels. A third may respond best to butyrophenone preparations which, via an inhibitory feedback circuit in the caudate loop, selectively decrease the responsivity of the caudal portion of the reticular formation, produce a dopamine-receptor blockade (Rossum, 1965) and, possibly by occupying GABA receptors, makes them inaccessible to glutamic acid. In this frame of reference, it is the differential, rather than the common, characteristics of the various groups of neuroleptics which are stressed to achieve a psychopharmacologically based diagnostic classification (Ban, 1969a). Needless to say, to date, all the efforts of grouping schizophrenics on the basis of the similarity of their response patterns to various neuroleptics have failed. Whether they failed because the action mechanism of one neuroleptic drug just does not differ from the other sufficiently to allow for meaningful clinical differences or because of deficiency in our clinical criteria remains undecided.

Independent of this, there is the clinical observation that any particular patient may be unaffected by a special neuroleptic agent, yet the same patient may respond to another neuroleptic drug. One possible explanation for this difference would be that different patients metabolize one or another neuroleptic differently. Obviously, the finding of any anomalous metabolism might provide a means of understanding why some patients are drug-responders while others are drug-refractory. But studies in this direction remained unrevealing (Curry *et al.*, 1970a; Curry *et al.*, 1970b; Green and Forrest, 1966). Another possibility considered was that the biochemical changes induced by neuroleptics differ from one patient to another. Nevertheless, systematic studies until recently* could not demonstrate any direct connnection between changes in 5-hydroxyindoleacetic acid

---

*A significant positive correlation between changes in 5-HIAA excretion in urine and therapeutic effects with thioproperazine was found by Albert *et al.* (1970). On the other hand, no correlation between 5-HIAA excretion and extrapyramidal signs was observed by the same authors.

In a recent study by Jus, it was found that when schizophrenics were given methionine, the concentration of methylated products, dimethyltryptamine and dimethyl-serotonin, rose significantly. The rise seemed to be correlated with the exacerbation of psychopathology (Kety, 1971).

(5-HIAA) and/or vanilmandelic acid (VMA) excretion and therapeutic effects either during treatment with reserpine or during treatment with chlorpromazine. Instead, a relationship between the changes in the principal urinary metabolites of serotonin and of the catecholamines on the one hand and the side-effects induced by reserpine and/or chlorpromazine were revealed. The main relationships were those between (a) a decrease in VMA and hypotensive manifestations, (b) an increase in 5-HIAA and gastroenteral and respiratory side-effects, and (c) an increase in homovanillic acid (HVA) and akinetic or akinetic-hypertonic extrapyramidal phenomena.

BRIDGING THE GAP

In view of the absence of well-defined biochemical, neurophysiological and clinical criteria in the differentiation of drug-responsive and drug-refractory schizophrenic patients, attempts are being made to use the conditioning method for this purpose. By the conditioning method, conditional reflex activity is studied, i.e. a behaviorally measurable activity which reflects demonstrable patterns of functioning in the central nervous system (Pavlov, 1928; Gastaut, 1957; Ban, 1964). A practical advantage of this method is that it can be employed equally in man and animal, and it is one of the very few methods which enables the investigator to study the same experimental variables in both species. Application of this method provides for a direct comparison of drug-action profiles in animals and psychopathological profiles in man. Nevertheless, our own work in this area of research has been restricted to humans, normal (i.e. physiological) and abnormal (i.e. psychopathological).

First Series of Studies

In the first phase of our studies, the Verdun Conditioning Procedure (VCP) was developed in the course of psychopathological studies which aimed to establish functionally based measurable correlates of psychopathological manifestations (Ban, Lehmann and Green, 1970). In the actual procedure, which was based on the classical conditioning paradigm, nonverbal stimuli were administered as conditional (visual) and unconditional (auditory) stimuli, and the responses to these stimuli were recorded in terms of changes in galvanic skin resistance (GSR) responses.

The VCP consisted of a 40-minute test procedure in the course of which eighty-six stimuli were given and eight psychophysiological functions were measured, i.e. startle response (SR), extinction of the orienting reflex (OR), unconditional reflex (UR), acquisition of conditional reflex (CR), extinction of conditional reflex (Ext), disinhibition of extinguished reflex (Dis), conditional stimulus differentiation (Diff) and conditional stimulus reversal (Rev) (Table XIV).

Since the VCP proved to be sensitive enough to differentiate among traditional clinical categories (Ban and Lehmann, 1971), the hypothesis was formulated that therapeutic responsiveness to phenothiazines (chlorpromazine, trifluoperazine, perphenazine, thioridazine and methotrimeprazine) can be predicted on the basis of pretreatment and short-term (two to four weeks) treatment performances on the VCP in schizophrenics. This was tested in a comprehensive clinical study on 120 patients. It was found that medium or high performance scores on SR, OR, Dis, Diff, mobility (Rev) and/or internal inhibition (Diff and mobility) predicted positive therapeutic changes in six months (at the 0.001 level of confidence). Furthermore, if no change in the excitatory process (acquisition) and/or internal inhibition scores occurred after four weeks of treatment with phenothiazines, this was predictive of a favorable therapeutic outcome in six months. Also, the preservation of Dis, Diff and Rev alone, or together with a decrease in the SR (which initially had been excessive), after four weeks of treatment indicated a potential for positive therapeutic changes (at the 0.001 level of confidence). Thus, by employing the conditioning method, it was possible to differentiate between two pharmacologically different schizophrenic populations, i.e. a phenothiazine-responsive and a phenothiazine-refractory group.

In the same study, the association between a well-preserved inhibitory process activity, as seen in both external (SR and Dis) and internal (Diff and mobility) inhibitory functions, and the therapeutic responsiveness to neuroleptics was substantiated with a high level of probability. This would suggest that the state of the inhibitory process (an inferred mechanism which constitutes various measurable functions such as Ext, Diff, Dis, etc.), including both external and internal inhibition, is a reliable indicator of potential responsiveness to psychopharmacological agents in schizophrenic patients. Thus it seems that the predrug impairment of inhibitory process, varying

TABLE XIV

THE VERDUN CONDITIONING PROCEDURE

I	Orienting period (SR and OR)	W	R	R	W	R	W	W	R	R	W	R	W	T	W
II	Conditioning process (CR)	WT	WT	W	WT	W	WT	WT	WT	W	WT	WT	WT	W	WT
III	Extinction process (Ext and Dis)	W	W	W	W	W	W	W	S	W	W				
IV	Differentiation period (Diff)	R	WT	WT	R	WT	R	WT	WT	R	WT	WT	R	WT	R
V	Reversal period	W	RT	RT	W	RT	RT	W	W	RT	R	W	RT	W	R
VI	US presentations (UR)	T	T	T											

W, white light; R, red light; T, tone; S, loud sound.

from patient to patient in schizophrenics provides for a *disease-specific* characteristic important in the prediction of therapeutic outcome with some of the presently available neuroleptic phenothiazines. Furthermore, the finding that no change in the excitatory process and/or internal inhibition scores after four weeks of treatment with phenothiazines was predictive of a favorable therapeutic outcome in six months suggested that there is also another predictive factor in operation. The *nonspecific* predictor variable which is the result of the drug-organism interaction seems to be independent of the disease-specific predictive variable, although it is of course possible, though unlikely on the basis of other experimental evidence, that the suppression of conditioning variables is a phenomenon resulting only from the natural history of the disease.

Attempts to correlate performance on the disease-specific predictive variables with performance profiles of the VCP in the clinical groups of schizophrenics failed. The psychopharmacologically homogeneous two groups cut across the traditional clinical categories. Thus by employing our conditioning method, the characterization of schizophrenic patients was meaningfully supplemented.

In spite of some indications, drug-specific predictive variables could not be identified in the course of our first series of experiments. In order to study this aspect, the VCP had to be extended into a battery of conditioning procedures.

Second Series of Studies

The Verdun Conditioning Battery utilizes seven conditioning techniques (i.e. GSR and Salivary Secretion, autonomic; Eyelid Closure and Defensive Finger Withdrawal, skeletomuscular; Ivanov-Smolensky's test for Generalization; modification of Astrup's Word Association Test for Differentiation; and Lehmann's Active Avoidance Test for Delay) and measures 8 psychophysiological functions which are expressed in terms of 11 experimental variables (Ban and Lehmann, 1971; Ban, Lehmann and Saxena, 1970).

Employing the VCB, we succeeded in obtaining significant differences in performance profiles between a normal and a chronically hospitalized psychotic population (Table XV). The functional ability to extinguish the autonomic orienting reflex was seen to be significantly impaired in the chronic hospitalized psychotic group, to-

TABLE XV

SIGNIFICANT DIFFERENCES BETWEEN NORMALS AND CHRONIC
PSYCHOTIC PATIENTS AT THE TIME OF FIRST TESTING
AND RETESTING

Variables	First Test Level of Significance (χ^2 test)	Retest Level of Significance (χ^2 test)
Autonomic		
Startle response	NS	NS
Orienting reflex	0.05	0.05
Acquisition of CR	NS	NS
Extinction of CR	NS	NS
Skeletomuscular		
Startle response	NS	NS
Orienting reflex	NS	NS
Acquisition of CR	0.01	NS
Extinction of CR	NS	NS
Generalization	0.001	0.001
Differentiation	0.001	0.001
Delay	0.001	0.001

gether with impairment of "integrational" functions such as generalization, differentiation, and delay (Ban, Lehmann and Saxena, 1970). This was followed by an attempt to construct a psychophysiological (conditioning) classification of chronic schizophrenia on the basis of four consecutive testings: once prior to drug (phenothiazine) withdrawal and three times afterwards within a one-year period. While our findings gave further substantiation to the nosological concept of schizophrenia, it also revealed the heterogeneity within the chronic schizophrenic population. This heterogeneity was reflected in the differential drug-withdrawal effects as well as in the finding that our schizophrenic population falls unto a hypothetical continuum. Quantitative analysis revealed that the mean total performance of the group of patients who could be maintained without medication for at least a period of one year was the highest (5.5) and the mean performance of the groups of patients who could not be maintained without medication for even a one-month period was the lowest (3.4) at the initial testing. The mean total performance of the group which could be maintained without medication for a period of eight months was only slightly lower (5.4) than that of the group which could be maintained without medication over the entire experimental period; and the mean total performance of the group which could not be maintained without medication for eight months was slightly higher (4.2) than that of the group which could not be maintained without medication for even a one-month period (Ban, Ananth and Lehmann, 1970).

Further qualitative analysis of our conditioning data uncovered two important phenomena, regression and dissociation, characteristically present in virtually all of our chronic schizophrenic patients. It was recognized that in all groups, performance in the autonomic functional system was the best and in the integrational functional system the worst, with performance in the skeletomuscular system being in between. Since among the three functional systems, the autonomic functional system is at the lowest level of organization and the integrational functional system at the highest, our findings suggest a characteristic regression from a higher to a lower level in a hierarchy of functioning in schizophrenic patients. Probably even more important was the finding that there were categories (combination of functions) in the experimental population which, at least in our experience, are not commonly encountered in normal subjects or in nonschizophrenic patients. These categories were characterized by dissociation, either within an individual functional system or between different functional systems. In normal subjects and other psychopathological groups, if there is no response to the first stimulus, there is no response to subsequent indifferent stimulus administrations. In our chronic schizophrenic population, however, there were four definite categories, two in the autonomic and two in the skeletomuscular functional system, in which the absence of SR was associated with either an extinguishable or an unextinguishable OR. Furthermore, when comparing the functional ability of the autonomic and skeletomuscular systems, we found a characteristic dissociation of functioning in the experimental population. This dissociation was manifest in the relatively well maintained functional ability of the autonomic functional system, in contrast to the impaired functional ability of the skeletomuscular functional system. The finding that the autonomic reflex may persist while the skeletomuscular is absent is consistent with Gantt's (1957) findings of a "split characterized by the persistence of one activity in the absence of the other." This split, he suggested, represents a maladaptation, a kind of built-in lack of integration of physiological systems. He named this phenomenon schizokinesis.

In a Pavlovian frame of reference, it was noted that in our chronic schizophrenic population, there was a shift in the equilibrium between excitatory- and inhibitory-process activity in the direction of inhibitory-process activity in patients who could be maintained without medication over a 12-month period (excitatory-process score/inhibitory-process score = 0.8) and in the direction of excitatory-process activity (excitatory-process score/inhibitory-process score = 1.2) in patients who could not be maintained without medication.

While our studies in establishing the psychopathological profiles of chronic schizophrenic patients in terms of conditional reflex variables has been in progress, Traugott and her collaborators (1968) have described the conditional reflex profile of chlorpromazine in animals as well as the effects of chlorpromazine, in terms of conditional reflex phenomena, in humans; and Saarma (1970) has described the conditional reflex profile of certain schizophrenic groups and also the effect of a number of neuroleptics on conditional reflex phenomena.

Whether the conditioning method will fill the gap between pharmacology and psychiatry is far from being answered. Nevertheless, in a recent report, Saarma and Vasar (1970) found that the therapeutic action of nicotinic acid was characterized by a positive effect on internal inhibition, seen in a decrease in the number of inadequate responses on a Word Association Test and in improved differentiation on a Motor Reflex Test. This effect of nicotinic acid is different from the action of neuroleptics which have an effect also on excitatory process activity, i.e. interfere with pathological conditional reflexes in schizophrenics. It is possible that this nicotinic-acid-responsive schizophrenic group consists of patients with dominant inhibitory process activity, i.e. patients in whom phenothiazine medication could be withdrawn—in our studies—without relapse. The differential action of nicotinic acid and neuroleptic drugs may also explain the therapeutic effects of nicotinic acid in some patients whose improvement on phenothiazines alone has reached a plateau (Kassay and Pinter, 1969).

Theoretical Considerations

Until the gap between pharmacology and psychiatry can be bridged, clinical psychopharmacological research will remain essentially the testing of a variety of hypotheses based on neurochemical theories which seem to be relevant to psychopathology in general or to certain behavioral manifestations in particular.

From a psychopharmacological point of view, most systematically explored are the hypotheses which implicate that a disorder of tryptophan and/or phenylalanine metabolism is involved in schizophrenic psychopathology. More recently, however, the transmethylation hypothesis of schizophrenia is gaining increasing importance.

Tryptophan Metabolism

The role of tryptophan metabolites in general and serotonin (5-hydroxytryptamine-5HT) in particular in the various clinical psychopathologies was summarized by Benda (1959), Smythies (1960), Sprince (1961) and more recently by Garattini and Valzelli (1965). While serotonin levels in the majority of schizophrenic patients were found to be within normal limits, there was at least one subgroup in which high values of serotonin (in the platelets) had been observed (Pare, Sandler and Stacey, 1958). Similarly, while urinary concentrations remained unchanged in the majority of schizophrenics (Rodnight, 1956), there was at least one subgroup of patients that was characterized by decreased urinary 5-HT excretion (Fischer, *et al.*, 1961). On the other hand, in the study of the urinary excretion of 5-hydroxyindoleacetic acid, the end product of serotonin catabolism, three groups of schizophrenics could be clearly differentiated on the basis of normal, decreased or increased urinary elimination of this substance. These three groups did not correspond to the traditional schizophrenic subcategories, although a consistently increased excretion was demonstrated in a group of catatonic schizophrenic patients by Buscaino and Stefanachi (1958). Other alterations in the urinary excretion of hydroxyindoles in schizophrenics are that in general, more indoles, and particularly hydroxyindoles, are detected in the urine of patient groups than in normal control groups, and that schizophrenics may excrete 6-hydroxyskatole.

Among the various hypotheses that tryptophan metabolites are involved in one way or another in schizophrenic psychopathology, the serotonin hypothesis of schizophrenia was chronologically first. It was put forward by Gaddum (1954) and by Woolley and Shaw (1954), based on the pharmacological antagonism between LSD_{25} and 5-HT. Subsequently they suggested that serotonin deficiency was in the background of the psychopathological changes in schizophrenic patients. This, however, was contradicted by the findings that administration of 5-hydroxytryptophan (5-HTP), the precursor of 5-HT, did not significantly change (improve) the behavior of schizophrenic patients and that the administration of reserpine, a *Rauwolfia* alkaloid which depletes brain serotonin levels, did not aggravate but did alleviate schizophrenic psychopathological symptoms (Brodsky, 1970). Hence the possibility was raised that not deficiency of serotonin but rather excess of serotonin would be responsible for the psychopathological changes seen in schizophrenic patients (Woolley, 1962). However, neither cinanserin, an antiserotonin substance (Gallant and Bishop, 1968), nor p-chlorophenylalanine, a specific blocker of the enzymatic hydroxylation of tryptophan preventing serotonin formation, displayed neuroleptic effects. Findings with α-methyldopa, a substance which interferes with 5-HT synthesis,* were less consistent (Pecknold *et al.*, 1971; St. Jean, Ban and Noe, 1965). Not only did α-methyldopa not improve schizophrenic psychopathological changes but in Herkert and Keup's (1969) study, it produced clinical deterioration in seven out of ten schizophrenic patients. In the latter study, the amount of tryptamine excretion seemed to be correlated with the severity of the psychiatric changes.

Besides serotonin, dimethylated tryptamine and serotonin metabolites have also been considered to play a role in the production of schizophrenic psychopathology. Fabing and Hawkins (1956) suggested that N, N-dimethyl-5-hydroxytryptamine (bufotenin) may evoke psychotic behavior in healthy humans. This was soon confirmed in a series of systematic studies (Arnold and Hofmann, 1957; Rosenberg, Isbell and Miner, 1963; Sai-Halasz, Brunecker and Szara, 1958; Szara, 1956). These findings were supplemented with more recent discoveries in which it was demonstrated that there is a decrease of nicotinic acid and N-methyl-pyridine-5-carboxamide ex-

*The inhibition of decarboxylase enzyme system by α-methyldopa results in not only a lowering of dopamine but also a lowering of serotonin concentration in the brain lasting for about 18 hours after the administration of the substance (Hess *et al.*, 1961).

cretion together with an increase in tryptamine, 3-indoleacetic acid and 5-hydroxyindoleacetic acid excretion in acute or exacerbated schizophrenics (Brune and Himwich, 1963; Brune and Pscheidt, 1961). In view of these findings, Brune (1967) formulated the hypothesis that, at least in some schizophrenic patients, there is a blockage within the kynurenine pathway of tryptophan metabolism (the metabolic path which results in the biological formation of nicotinic acid) which in turn leads to increased tryptophan metabolism along the other two possible pathways—the tryptamine pathway, with the end-product of 3-indoleacetic acid, and the serotonin pathway, with the end-product of 5-hydroxyindoleacetic acid, (Faurbye, 1968). It was speculated that interference with the biological formation of nicotinic acid may be responsible, at least in part, for the excess of available methyl groups and that the reaction of these methyl groups with the increased indole metabolites results in the formation of the dimethylated psychotoxic metabolic products (Fig. 20). That dimethylated psychotoxic metabolites can, in fact, be formed in the mammalian organism from tryptamine and 5-hydroxytryptamine was first demonstrated by Axelrod (1961), who isolated an enzyme which has this function from the lung of rabbits and more recently,

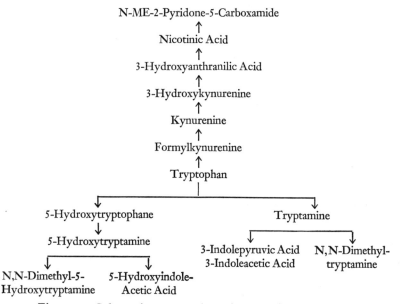

Figure 20. Schematic presentation of tryptophan metabolism.

by Mandell and Morgan (1970) who were able to show the presence of such an enzyme, more specific than Axelrod's lung enzyme, in the brains of man, rat and chick. However, until recently,* attempts to find dimethyltryptamine (DMT) in the urine of schizophrenic patients have failed (Feldstein, Hoagland and Freeman, 1961; Rodnight, 1956; Szara, 1967). But Bumpus and Page (1955) reported the occurrence of a bufotenin (dimethylated 5-hydroxytryptamine)-like substance in human urine, and Fischer *et al.* (1961) found the same substance present in the urine of twenty-five out of twenty-six hallucinating patients. Finally, Tanimukai *et al.* (1967) verified that bufotenin is present in excess in the urine of schizophrenics.† Nevertheless, the first attempt to obtain improvement in schizophrenic patients with a diet containing reduced amounts of both tryptophan and methionine remained unsuccessful (Berlet *et al.*, 1965, 1966), and at least one attempt to obtain improvement in schizophrenics by opening the kynurine pathway of metabolism by pyridoxine administration remained unconvincing (Ban and Lehmann, 1970).

Another hypothesis in which a disorder of tryptophan metabolism is implicated in schizophrenic psychopathology was put forward by Greiner and Nicholson (1965). They suggested that at least in certain schizophrenics, the normal route of melatonin synthesis from serotonin is blocked, presumably because of a congenital absence of O-methyltransferase, and consequently, instead of melatonin, hallucinogenic compounds like harmine are produced. In any event, since harmine itself is an O-methylated compound, the original Greiner-Nicholson hypothesis lacks cohesion (Smythies, 1967a). On the other hand, their prediction based on this hypothesis, that inhibiting the

*Most recently, Tanimukai *et al.* (1970) employed thin-layer chromatography and found N-methylserotonin, N, N-dimethyltryptamine and 5-methoxy-N, N-dimethyltryptamine in the urine of schizophrenics, especially when patients were receiving tranylcypromine with or without cysteine.

†In their latest paper, Tanimukai *et al.* (1970) reported on bufotenin (4 to 10μg per 24 hours) both in free and conjugated forms in the urine of four schizophrenic patients under dietary control when they were receiving tranylcypromine, with or without cysteine loading. In the absence of monoamine oxidase blockade, bufotenin was also excreted in some patients but less than 1μg/day. Increase of urinary bufotenin and other N-methylated indoleamines were observed, however, about two weeks before the mental and behavioral symptoms of the schizophrenic patients worsened and these elevated levels continued during the period of behavioral exacerbation.

copper-dependent enzyme tyrosinase by means of a low-copper diet plus penicillamine administration should alleviate schizophrenic symptoms,* was confirmed in at least one clinical study carried out in a metabolic unit (Greiner, 1970). Clinical findings in other studies carried out under less well controlled conditions, however, remained inconsistent (Affleck *et al.*, 1969; Hollister *et al.*, 1966).

Phenylalanine Metabolism

Among the various hypotheses that phenylalanine metabolites are involved in one way or another in schizophrenic psychopathology, the norepinephrine hypothesis of schizophrenia was chronologically first. Accordingly, it was suggested that an excess of NE concentration in the brain was in the background of the psychopathological changes in schizophrenic patients. This, however, was contradicted by the findings that administration of α-methyl-p-tyrosine, a specific tyrosine hydroxylase inhibitor which reduces NE levels without decreasing 5-HT concentrations, did not significantly change (improve) the behavior of schizophrenic patients and that the administration of disulfiram, a dopamine-β-hydroxylase inhibitor which decreases the synthesis of NE, did not alleviate but did aggravate schizophrenic psychopathological symptoms (Charalampous and Brown, 1967; Gershon *et al.*, 1967; Goldstein *et al.*, 1964; Heath *et al.*, 1965; Musacchio, Kopin and Snyder, 1964). Hence the possibility was raised that not the excess of NE but rather the increase of dopamine concentration would be responsible for the psychopathological changes seen in schizophrenic patients. This contention was supported by the finding that administration of l'dopa, the precursor of dopamine, did produce aggravation of psychopathological symptoms in schizophrenics. In favor of the hypothesis that dopamine is involved in the pathogenesis of schizophrenia is that all active neuroleptics of the phenothiazine and the butyrophenone category antagonize some of the central effects of dopamine (Domino, 1969).

*Greiner and Nicholson (1965) found that obstructing the increased melanogenesis produced clinical improvement in "patients' negative symptoms of schizophrenia but not much change in positive symptoms." According to them, blocking melanin formation does not decrease the production of hallucinogenic harmala alkaloids. On the other hand, chlorpromazine inhibits serotonin production and consequently decreases the formation of psychotoxic harmala alkaloids. On the basis of this, they suggested that "effective therapy in schizophrenia may be due to blocking the formation of melanin and inhibiting the synthesis of serotonin."

After Cannon had published his discovery (1915) on the role of adrenal hormones (norepinephrine and epinephrine) in the adaptation to "stress," the notion that abnormal mental states are the result of a "faulty adaptation" to "overwhelming" environmental stimulation was entertained by various psychiatric schools. Among the first were Osmond and Smythies (1952), who formulated the hypothesis that schizophrenia is the outcome of stress-induced anxiety and a failure of metabolism which results in highly toxic mescalin-like ("M") compounds. Harley-Mason (1952) suggested that 3,4-dimethoxy-phenylethylamine (DMPEA) is the toxic agent responsible for the psychopathological changes and put forward the hypothesis that the production of DMPEA (in the adrenals) is the result of "transmethylation," in which the physiological N-methylation of norepinephrine to epinephrine is replaced by the pathological O-methylation of the phenol ring of dopamine. In favor of this hypothesis was the early finding that DMPEA in animal studies induced "experimental catatonia" (deJong, 1931; Noteboom, 1934). An alternative hypothesis, that adrenochrome, a psychotoxic oxidation product of epinephrine (Fig. 21) is the "M" substance, was suggested by Hoffer, Osmond and Smythies (1954). Its production was thought to be the result of the increased phenolase (oxidase) activity of schizophrenic serum (Hoffer, 1958, 1964, 1966; Hoffer and Kenyon, 1957). That adrenochrome can be obtained by treating epinephrine with various oxidants (including inorganic) had been demonstrated long before the adrenochrome hypothesis of schizophrenia was formulated (Green and Richter, 1937).

In subsequent years, both the adrenochrome and the DMPEA hypotheses were systematically examined and scrutinized also by clinical psychopharmacological methods. Chronologically, at first some of the essential components of the adrenochrome (and/or adrenolutine) hypothesis were questioned. Only in selected groups of schizophrenics (acute and aggressive) was it possible to demonstrate a definite increment in urinary catecholamine excretion (Pscheidt, 1964; Kety, 1966), while essentially no difference in the excretion of epinephrine, norepinephrine and vanilmandelic acid between normal subjects and other schizophrenic patients could be found (Bergsman, 1959; La-Brosse, Mann and Kety, 1963; Mann and LaBrosse, 1959; Pind and Faurbye, 1961). The augmentation of oxidative processes remained,

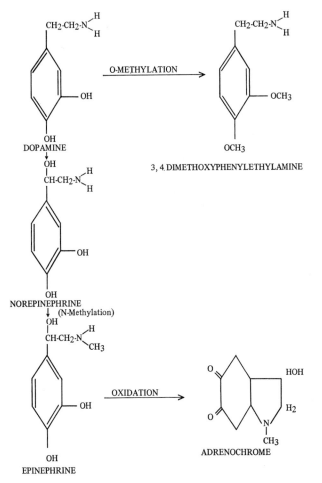

Figure 21. The formation of 3,4-dimethoxyphenylethylamine (DMPEA) from dopamine and the formation of adrenochrome from epinephrine.

at best, a controversial issue (Cohen *et al.*, 1958, 1959; Hoffer and Kenyon, 1957; LaBrosse, Mann and Kety, 1963; Leach and Heath, 1956), and the presence of adrenochrome (Hoffer, 1958; Osmond and Hoffer, 1966) or adrenolutin (Sulkowitch and Altschule, 1959) in plasma could not be confirmed by special techniques (Feldstein, 1959; Randrup and Munkvad, 1960; Szara, Axelrod and Perlin, 1958). After a considerable dispute (Schwartz, Jacobsen and Petersen, 1956; Taubmann and Jantz, 1957), however the psychotomimetic properties of adrenochrome were confirmed (Grof *et al.*, 1963). Nevertheless, direct evidence of a necessary enzyme which is capable of oxidizing epinephrine to adrenochrome could only be given *in vitro* (Axelrod, 1964). In clinical psychopharmacological studies, findings with high-dosage ascorbic acid administration—to prevent the formation of adrenochrome from epinephrine via the inhibition of ceruloplasmin and adrenaline oxidase (Hoffer and Osmond, 1963; McDonald, 1958, 1961) remained unconvincing; and the therapeutic effects obtained with d'penicillamine, which was suggested to increase the formation of 5,6-dihydroxy-N-methyl-indole from adrenochrome and decrease the formation of psychotoxic adrenolutine (Hoffer, 1958, 1960, 1964, 1966; Hoffer and Kenyon, 1957), were more likely related to another mechanism, i.e. blocking of melanin formation.

The DMPEA hypothesis gained new impetus in 1962, when Friedhoff and Van Winkle found a "pink spot" in the urine of acute schizophrenic patients. By chromatography, they identified the "pink spot" as 3,4-dimethoxyphenylethylamine (DMPEA), the para-O-methylation product of dopamine. Faurbye and Pind (1964), Perry Hansen and MacIntyre (1964), Perry *et al.* (1967) and Wagner *et al.* (1966), however failed to isolate this dimethylated dopamine metabolite from the urine of chronic schizophrenics, even after tritium-labeled dopamine, dopa or monoamine oxidase inhibitor administration (Faurbye, 1968); and Nishimure and Gjessing (1965) could not find it in the urine of a periodic catatonic patient. In the controversy* which arose, Takaseda *et al.* (1963), Studnitz and Nyman (1965) and Pue, Hoare and Adamson (1969) stated that they were able to identify the substance in both normals and schizophrenics, although the latter group had a statistically significant higher incidence of DMPEA among mental patients than in mentally "normal" controls. It was also suggested that the "pink spot," or spots (Watt *et al.*, 1969) is of dietary origin,† while Closs, Wad and Ose (1967)

*According to Feldstein (1970), counterclaims have been advanced that DMPEA is present in urine from neither schizophrenic nor normal subjects, that DMPEA is not an endogenous substance but is rather a dietary artifact, that DMPEA has been misidentified, that DMPEA is actually a mixture of several components, and that DMPEA is not specific for schizophrenia.

†The contention that the "pink spot" is due to tea consumption was not borne out by the application of "t" test (Friedhoff, 1970).

asserted that it is a metabolite of chlorpromazine (nor_2-chlorpromazine sulfoxide) related to the treatment of patients rather than to psychopathology. On the other hand, Friedhoff and Van Winkle's (1962) findings were confirmed by Kuehl (1967), Kuehl et al. (1964), Sen and McGreer (1964), and Stam, Heslinga and Tilburg (1969); and also by Bourdillon and Ridges (1967) in a controlled study. Furthermore, while Smythies and Sykes (1967) were able to demonstrate that DMPEA has an inhibitory action with a bimodal distribution on the conditioned avoidance response of the rat, resembling the effect of plasma protein fractions from schizophrenic patients on a mouse behavior test (Bergen et al., 1960), the substance failed to induce or precipitate psychopathological reactions in normal subjects or in schizophrenic patients in remission (Friedhoff and Hollister, 1966; Hollister and Friedhoff, 1966; Shulgin, Sargent and Naranjo, 1966). On the other hand, when administered to subjects pretreated with a monoamine oxidase inhibitor, DMPEA was shown to have psychotogenic effects (Feldstein, 1970).

Transmethylation Hypothesis

With these new data on phenylalanine and tryptophan metabolism, Harley-Mason's (1952) idea that transmethylation is the process which may be responsible for the formation of psychotoxic substances regained importance in Kety's (1961, 1966, 1967) formulation of the transmethylation hypothesis of schizophrenia. He shifted the emphasis from the psychotoxic compound produced by (Harley-Mason, 1952), or as a result of (Hoffer, 1964), transmethylation to the biochemical process itself. Accordingly, it was suggested that the disorder of the methylation process, a fundamental biochemical process whereby methyl groups are attached to compounds within the organism, is primarily responsible for the functional changes at both the neuronal and behavioral levels. The same disorder may also lead to the production of abnormally methylated compounds, e.g. DMT, bufotenin (Szara, 1961, Fischer et al. 1961) or DMPEA (Friedhoff and Van Winkle, 1962) which would aggravate the situation by adding their own psychotoxic effects to the neuronal functions already disordered by the abnormal transmethylating mechanism (Smythies, 1967a, b). Considering that transmethylation is an all-encompassing process which, among many others, is responsible for the formation of epinephrine from norepinephrine, melatonin from acetylserotonin, and N-methylnicotinamide from nicotinamide in the organism (Mahler and Cordes, 1966), it is conceivable to suggest that its disturbance may produce such diverse but fundamental and all-embracing changes as are encountered in schizophrenic patients.

In favor of the transmethylation hypothesis of schizophrenia are clinical findings with the administration of methionine sulphoximine (MSO). At first, Krakoff (1961) reported that MSO, an antimetabolite of methionine, if given to normal people in a dose over 200 mg/day, induced a "toxic" psychosis accompanied by EEG signs of an organic disturbance. Following this lead, Heath, Nesselhof and Timmons (1966) fed MSO to ten schizophrenic patients and nine prisoners who acted as controls. While none of the schizophrenic patients showed clinical worsening, some in fact showing an apparent alleviation of symptoms, all the controls given MSO reacted with psychotic manifestations. Similarly, the EEG was abnormal in all the controls and showed slow waves, whereas no abnormality was seen in the case of any of the schizophrenic patients. These findings support the hypothesis that in schizophrenics there is an "overactive" methylating enzymatic system which is made normal by the MSO, whereas in normals, methylation is reduced too much, producing a psychosis (Smythies, 1967a). Also in favor of the transmethylation hypothesis are Buscaino, Spadetta and Carella's (1966) findings. By incubating deproteinized blood with betaine as a methyldonor and nicotinamide as a methyl acceptor, they found a much greater increase in N-methylnicotinamide formation in the blood of "active" schizophrenic patients than in the blood of normal subjects or of patients with other psychopathological conditions. Probably most important, however, is the direct *in vivo* presentation of an abnormality of methylation in schizophrenics by Israelstam, Johnson and Winchell (1967). They administered 25μCi of ^{14}C–labeled methionine intravenously and monitored the $^{14}CO_2$ content of the expired air. In a group of normal subjects, they found a peak of $^{14}CO_2$ excretions after 18 to 25 minutes of ^{14}C–labeled methionine administration, followed by a gradual decline. In contrast to this, in the schizophrenic group there was a rising curve for a period of two and a half hours. These findings are consistent with the speculation that a rate-limiting, enzymatically based step is delaying the conversion of $^{14}CH_3$ to

$^{14}CO_2$ in schizophrenics, although the possibility of a larger methionine pool (or more specifically, transmethylating pool) could not be excluded. These findings were further qualified in subsequent studies by Israelstam and his collaborators (1970). It was revealed that $^{14}CO_2$ excretion in a group of schizophrenic patients in remission did not appear to be different from the normal and that only in the acute schizophrenic group (actively hallucinating) followed $^{14}CO_2$ excretion the pattern previously seen in schizophrenics. Distinctly different from the schizophrenic curve was the $^{14}CO_2$ curve of depressive patients in which an initial rapid rise in the rate of appearance of $^{14}CO_2$ reached an amplitude two or three times that observed in normal subjects and was followed by a rapid decrease.* It should also be noted that the recently isolated substance which causes the peculiar odor in the sweat of schizophrenic patients has been recognized as the result of transmethylation and identified as trans-3-methyl-2-hexenoic acid (Smith, Thompson and Koster, 1969). While the latter finding may, of course, support the transmethylation hypothesis of schizophrenia, it may also reflect the profoundness of a disturbance which affects approximately one percent of the world's population.

The active methyl donor involved in the transmethylation of amines is S-adenosylmethionine (SAMe) which is formed by the reaction of methionine and adenosine triphosphate in the presence of an activating enzyme in the liver (Cantoni, 1953; Axelrod, 1962). In more recent experiments, Baldessarini (1967) found an increase of SAMe levels in the central nervous system after methionine loading but a depletion (unloading via transmethylation) of the brain concentrations of SAMe after the administration of monoamine oxidase inhibitors (MAOI) which tend to mobilize methylation processes. These observations correspond to the clinical findings that schizophrenic patients given methyl donors—methionine or betaine—and a MAOI suffered a striking exacerbation of psychosis (Ananth et al., 1970; Alexander et al., 1963; Berlet et al., 1965; Brune and Himwich, 1962; Park, Baldessarini and Kety, 1965; Pollin, Cardon and Kety, 1961; Spaide et al., 1969; Sprince et al., 1963). Further-

---

*As seen from this discussion, there are various hypotheses regarding the nature of the methylation disorder in schizophrenia, e.g. overactive methylating enzymatic systems, a rate-limiting enzymatically based step which delays the conversion of methyl groups to carbon dioxide, and a larger (than normal) methionine pool.

more, they support the speculation that transmethylation could be facilitated by such simple means as increasing the availability of the methyl donor by methionine loading (Efron, 1965) and that transmethylation could be prevented or interfered with by such simple means as nicotinic acid administration (Kety, 1966).*

The speculation that transmethylation could be facilitated by such simple means as increasing the availability of the methyl donor by methionine loading was contested, however by Haydu *et al.* (1965). They argued that methionine-induced aggravation of psychopathology is related to excessive transmethylation in schizophrenics and suggested that methionine as a precursor of thiol groups produces an increased effort readiness without discharge, which results in aggravation of psychopathological symptoms. This hypothesis was supported by their findings that hydroxychloroquine, a substance which has the opposite effect to methionine on thiol groups, produced significant amelioration of schizophrenic symptoms.

The speculation that transmethylation could be prevented or interfered with by such simple means as nicotinic acid administration, a methyl acceptor substance, has remained undecided to date (Ban and Lehmann, 1970). In human pharmacological studies, however, the administration of megadosages, 3000 mg./day, of nicotinic acid did not reduce the stress-induced increase in the synthesis of methylated compounds, i.e. epinephrine and creatinine, a methylation product of guanidoacetic acid (Ellerbrook and Purdy, 1970). Nevertheless, the facts remain that parenteral administration of catechol-O-methyltransferase exacerbates the clinical symptoms of schizophrenia (Hall *et al.*, 1969) and also that all presently available phenothiazine and butyrophenone neuroleptics have an inhibitory action on the methyltransferase enzyme system (Buscaino, Spadetta and Carella, 1966), both of which findings are in favor of the transmethylation hypothesis of schizophrenia.

*In Baldessarini's experiments nicotinanide had no effect on SAMe levels.

Chapter 5

CONCLUDING REMARKS

THERE are numerous reports which suggest that schizophrenia and coeliac disease (gluten enteropathy) occur in the same individual more often than expected by chance. Coeliac disease is a hereditary disease, with marked psychic and somatic symptoms, which usually improve when wheat gluten and its analogues in other cereals are not eaten. The role of wheat glutens in schizophrenic psychopathology, however, was only recently demonstrated in a controlled clinical study by Dohan *et al.* (1969). They found that relapsed schizophrenics randomly assigned to a milk- and cereal-free diet on admission to a locked ward were transferred to an open ward considerably more rapidly than those assigned to a high-cereal diet. This difference, however, was eliminated by the addition of gluten to the diet of patients on the cereal-free "treatment" regime. Thus it seems that schizophrenic psychopathology can be modified and alleviated not only by adding to the diet a neuroleptic drug but also by eliminating from the diet certain dietary substances.

Since the introduction of chlorpromazine, the first neuroleptic drug, almost two decades have passed. In spite of all the changes which have been encountered during this period, schizophrenia in all the civilized countries in the world has remained one of the greatest public health problems, i.e. neuroleptics have not cured the schizophrenic patient. What neuroleptics have done, however, is separate the various "pathological" manifestations which are prone to environmental manipulations from those which cannot be affected by social "treatments" in schizophrenic patients.

How far the transmethylation hypothesis or any of the other hypotheses will lead us in solving the problem of schizophrenia, i.e. the psychopathological manifestations which are unaffected by environmental contingencies, it is impossible to know. These new hypotheses, however, are based on the new way of thinking about schizophrenia, which was brought about by chlorpromazine and the introduction of the pharmacological method to psychiatric problems.

The introduction of this pharmacological method has already led to a reassessment of instruments and points of reference in psychiatry. This is why we are talking about a revolution, a psychopharmacological revolution which will lead hopefully to a new understanding of the various mechanisms operating in schizophrenic patients.

BIBLIOGRAPHY

Achté, K.A.: The course of schizophrenic and schizophreniform psychoses. *Acta Psychiat. Neurol. Scand.*, supp. *155*, 1961.

Ackner, B. and Oldham, A.J.: Insulin treatment of schizophrenia. *Lancet*, *1*:504-506, 1962.

Adelson, D. and Epstein, L.J.: A study of phenothiazines with male and female chronically ill schizophrenic patients. *J. Nerv. Ment. Dis.*, *134*:543-554, 1962.

Affleck, J.W., Cooper, A.J., Forrest, A.D., Smythies, J.R. and Zealley, A.K.: Penicillamine and schizophrenia—a clinical trial. *Brit. J. Psychiat.*, *115*:173-176, 1969.

Albert, J.M., Palaic, D., Tetreault, L., Panisset, J.C., Dhaiti, G. and Desaty, J.: Effect of thioproperazine on 5-HIAA content in urine and cerebrospinal fluid of chronic schizophrenic patients. *Dis. Nerv. Syst.*, *31*(11):140-144, 1970.

Alexander, F., Curtis, G.C., Sprince, H. and Crosley, A.P.: L-methionine and l-tryptophan feedings in non-psychotic and schizophrenic patients with and without tranylcypromine. *J. Nerv. Ment. Dis.*, *137*:135-142, 1963.

Ananth, J.V., Ban, T.A., Lehmann, H.E. and Bennett, Jean: Nicotinic acid in the prevention and treatment of methionine-induced exacerbation of psychopathology in schizophrenics. *Canad. Psychiat. Assn. J.*, *15*:3-14, 1970.

Arnold, O.H. and Hofmann, G.: Zur Psychopathologie des Dimethyltryptamine: ein weiterer Beitrag zur Pharmakopsychiatrie: vorlaufige Mitteilung. *Wien. Z. Nervenheilk*, *13*:438-445, 1957.

Ashcroft, G.W., MacDougall, E.J. and Barker, P.A.: A comparison of tetrabenazine and chlorpromazine in chronic schizophrenia. *J. Ment. Sci.*, *107*:287-293, 1961.

Astrup, C.: *Schizophrenia: Conditional Reflex Studies*. Springfield, Thomas, 1962.

Auch, W.: Beeinflusst die Psychopharmakotherapie die Aufnahmeentwicklung, die stationare Behandlungsdauer und den Verlauf endogener Psychosen? *Fortschr. Neurol Psychiat.*, *31*:548-564, 1963.

Axelrod, J.: Enzymatic formation of psychomimetic metabolites from normally occurring compounds. *Science, 134*:343-344, 1961.

Axelrod, J.: The enzymatic N-methylation of serotonin and other amines. *J. Pharmacol. Exp. Ther., 138*:28-33, 1962.

Axelrod, J.: Enzymatic oxidation of epinephrine to adrenochrome by the salivary gland. *Biochem. Biophys. Acta, 85*:247-254, 1964.

Ayd, F.J. Jr.: Fluphenazine: twelve years' experience. *Dis. Nerv. Syst., 29*:744-747, 1968.

Azima, H., Durost, H. and Arthurs, D.: The effect of R-1625 (Halo-peridol) in mental syndromes: a multiblind study. *Amer. J. Psychiat., 117*:546-547, 1960.

Baker, A.A., Game, J.A. and Thorpe, J.G.: Physical treatment for schizophrenia. *J. Ment. Sci., 104*:860-864, 1958.

Baldessarini, R.J.: Factors influencing S-adenosyl-methionine levels in mammalian tissues. In Himwich, H.E., Kety, S.S. and Smythies, J.R. (Eds.): *Amines and Schizophrenia.* Oxford, Pergamon Press, 1967.

Ban, T.A.: Clinical studies on the antipsychotic properties of haloperidol versus permitil. Symposium Internazionale Sull' Haloperidol e Tri-peridol, Instituto Luso Farmaco d'Italia, Milan, 1962.

Ban, T.A.: *Conditioning and Psychiatry.* Chicago, Aldine, 1964.

Ban, T.A.: The butyrophenones in psychiatry. In Lehmann, H.E. and Ban, T.A. (Eds.): *The Butryrophenones in Psychiatry.* Montreal, Quebec Psychopharmacological Research Association, 1964.

Ban, T.A.: Human pharmacology and systematic clinical studies with a new phenothiazine. In Jenner, F.A. (Ed): *Leeds Symposium on Behavioral Disorders.* Essex, Vernon Lock, 1965.

Ban, T.A.: *Psychopharmacology.* Baltimore, Williams and Wilkins, 1969a.

Ban, T.A.: Treatment of acute and chronic psychoses with haloperidol. Review of clinical results. *Curr. Ther. Res., 11*:284-288, 1969b.

Ban, T.A.: Psychopharmacology and psychiatric practice in the seventies. A personal view. *Canada. Ment. Health, 19*(1):8-12, 1971.

Ban, T.A., Ananth, J.V. and Lehmann, H.E.: Conditioning in the prediction of drug withdrawal effects in chronic schizophrenic patients. Presented at the Meeting of the Collegium Internationale Neuro-Psychopharmacologicum, Prague, Czechoslovakia, 1970.

Ban, T.A., Ferguson, K. and Lehmann, H.E.: The effect of clopenthixol on chronic psychiatric patients (clinical note). *Amer. J. Psychiat., 119*:984-985, 1963.

Ban, T.A. and Lehmann, H.E.: Efficacy of haloperidol in drug refractory patients. *Int. J. Neuropsychiat., 3*:79-86, 1967.

Ban, T.A. and Lehmann, H.E.: Nicotinic acid in the treatment of schizophrenia. Toronto, Canadian Mental Health Association, 1970.

Ban, T.A. and Lehmann, H.E.: *Experimental Approaches to Psychiatric Diagnosis.* Springfield, Thomas, 1971.

Ban, T.A., Lehmann, H.E. and Green, A.A.: Conditional reflex variables in the prediction of therapeutic responsiveness to phenothiazines in the schizophrenias. In Wittenborn, J.R., Goldberg, S.C. and May, P.R.A. (Eds.): *Psychopharmacology and the Individual Patient.* Hewlett, Raven Press, 1970.

Ban, T.A., Lehmann, H.E. and Saxena, B.M.: A conditioning test battery for the study of psychopathological mechanisms and psychopharmacological effects. *Canad. Psychiat. Assn. J.,* 15 (3):301-308, 1970.

Ban, T.A., Lehmann, H.E., Sterlin, C. and Saxena, B.M.: Predictors of therapeutic responsivity to thiothixene. In Cerletti, A. and Bové, F.J. (Eds.): *The Present Status of Psychotropic Drugs.* Basel, Excerpta Medica Foundation, 1969.

Ban, T.A., Papathomopulos, E. and Schwarz, L.: Clinical studies with thioproperazine (Majeptil). *Comp. Psychiat.,* 3:289-291, 1962.

Ban, T.A. and Schwarz, L.: Systematic studies with levomepromazine. *J. Neuropsychiat.,* 5:112-117, 1963.

Ban, T.A. and Stonehill, E.: Clinical observations on the differential effects of a butyrophenone (haloperidol) and a phenothiazine (fluphenazine) in chronic schizophrenic patients. In Lehmann, H.E. and Ban, T.A. (Eds.): *The Butyrophenones in Psychiatry.* Montreal, Quebec Psychopharmacological Research Association, 1964.

Bankier, R.G., Pettit, D.E. and Bergen, B.: A comparative study of fluphenazine enanthate and trifluoperazine in chronic schizophrenic patients. *Dis. Nerv. Syst.,* 29:56-61, 1968.

Bannister, D., Salmon, P. and Leiberman, D.M.: Diagnosis-treatment relationships in psychiatry: a statistical analysis. *Brit. J. Psychiat.,* 110:726-732, 1964.

Bartolucci, G., Lehmann, H.E., Ban, T.A. and Lee, H.: Clinical studies with clopenthixol (Sordinol) on chronic psychiatric patients. *Curr. Ther. Res.,* 8:581-584, 1966.

Battegay, R. and Gehring, A.: Vergleichende Untersuchungen an Schizophrenen der Preneuroleptischen und der Postneuroleptischen Era. *Pharmakopsychiat. Neuro-Psychopharm.,* 1(2):107-112, 1968.

Benda, P. (1959): In Garattini, S. and Valzelli, L. (Eds): *Serotonin.* Amsterdam, Elsevier, 1965.

Bergen, J.R., Pennell, R.B., Freeman, H. and Hoagland, H.: Rat behavior changes in response to a blood factor from normal and psychotic persons. *Arch. Neurol.*, 2:146-150, 1960.

Bergsman, A.: The urinary excretion of adrenaline and noradrenaline in some mental diseases. A clinical and experimental study. *Acta Psychiat. Neurol. Scand.*, suppl., 133, 1959.

Berlet, H.H., Brill, C., Himwich, H.E., Kohl, H., Matsumoto, K., Pscheidt, G.R., Spaide, J., Tourlentes, T.T. and Valverde, G.M.: Effect of diet on schizophrenic behavior. In Hoch, P. and Zubin, J. (Eds.): *Psychopathology of Schizophrenia.* New York, Grune and Stratton, 1966.

Berlet, H.H., Matsumoto, K., Pscheidt, G.R., Spaide, J., Bull, C. and Himwich, H.E.: Biochemical correlates of behavior in schizophrenic patients. Schizophrenic patients receiving tryptophan and methionine or methionine together with a monoamine oxidase inhibitor. *Arch. Gen. Psychiat. 13*:521-531, 1965.

Bertolotti, P. and Munarini, D.: Therapeutic experiences in neuropsychiatry with a derivative of benzoquinolizine (RO 1-9569). *Riv. Sper. Freniat., 85*:185-193, 1961.

Bishop, M. P., Fulmer, T.E. and Gallant, D.M.: Thiothixene versus trifluoperazine in newly-admitted schizophrenic patients. *Curr. Ther. Res., 8*:509-514, 1966.

Bishop, M.P., Gallant, D.M. and Sykes, T.F.: Extrapyramidal side effects and therapeutic response. *Arch. Gen. Psychiat., 13*:155-162, 1965.

Bishop, M.P., Mason, L.B., Gallant, D.M. and Bishop, G.: One year trial of the antipsychotic acridan compound SK&F 14336. *Curr. Ther. Res., 11*(7):447-455, 1969.

Blackburn, H.L. and Allen, J.L.: Behavioral effects of interrupting and resuming tranquilizing medication among schizophrenics. *J. Nerv. Ment. Dis., 133*:303-308, 1961.

Bleuler, E.P., (1911): Dementia Praecox and the Group of Schizophrenias. (trans. Zinkin, J.). New York, International Universities Press, 1950.

Bloom, J.B., Davis, N. and Wecht, C.H.: Effect on the liver of long-term tranquilizing medication. *Amer. J. Pschiat., 121*:788-797, 1965.

Bobon, D.P., Debroye, A., Goffioul, L. and Pinchard, A.: Le pimozide, 16 mois de follow-up. *Acta Neurol. Belg., 68*:887-894, 1968.

Bobon, J., Collard, J., Pinchard, A., Bobon, D.P. and Debroye, A.: Neuroleptiques à longue durée d'action. II. Etude pilote du pimozide (R 6238). *Acta Neurol. Belg., 68*:137-153, 1968.

Bohacek, N.: Pharmakogene depressive Verschiebung bei schizophrenen Psychosen. *A. Prav. Med., 10*:511, 1965.

Bolt, A.G. and Forrest, I.S.: Metabolic studies of chlorpromazine induced hyperpigmentation of the skin in psychiatric patients. *Agressologie*, *9*:1-6, 1968.

Bookhammer, R.S., Meyers, R.W., Schober, C.C. and Piotrowski, Z.A.: A five year clinical follow up study of schizophrenics treated by Rosen's "Direct Analysis" compared with controls. *Amer. J. Psychiat.*, *123*(5):602-604, 1966.

Borowski, T. and Tolwinsi, T.: Treatment of paranoid schizophrenics with chlorpromazine and group therapy. *Dis. Nerv. Syst.*, *30*:201-202, 1969.

Bourdillon, R.E. and Ridges, A.P.: The pink spot. *Lancet*, *1*:429-430, 1966.

Bowers, M.B., Jr. and Astrachan, B.M.: Depression in acute schizophrenic psychosis. *Amer. J. Psychiat.*, *123*(8):976-979, 1967.

Brill, H. and Patton, R.E.: Analysis of 1955-56 population fall in New York State Mental Hospitals in first year of large-scale use of tranquilizing drugs. *Amer. J. Psychiat. 114*:509-517, 1957.

Brill, H. and Patton, R.E.: Analysis of population reduction in New York State Mental Hospitals during the first four years of large-scale therapy with psychotropic drugs. *Amer. J. Psychiat.*, *116*:495-509, 1959.

Brill, H. and Patton, R.E.: Clinical-statistical analysis of population changes in New York State Mental Hospitals since introduction of psychotropic drugs. *Amer. J. Psychiat.*, *119*:20-35, 1962.

Brodsky, L.: A biochemical survey of schizophrenia. *Canad. Psychiat. Assn. J.*, *15*(4):375-388, 1970.

Brophy, J.J.: Single daily doses of neuroleptic drugs. *Dis. Nerv. Syst.*, *30*:120-123, 1969.

Brugmans, J.: A multicentric clinical evaluation of pimozide: preliminary report. *Acta Neurol. Psychiat. Belg. 68*:875, 1968.

Brune, G.G.: Tryptophan metabolism in psychoses. In Himwich, H.E., Kety, S.S. and Smythies, J.R. (Eds): *Amines and Schizophrenia*. Oxford, Pergamon Press, 1967.

Brune, G.G. and Himwich, H.E.: Effects of methionine loading on the schizophrenic patients. *J. Nerv. Ment. Dis.*, *134*:447-450, 1962.

Brune, G.G. and Himwich, H.E.: Biogenic amines and behavior in schizophrenic patients. In Wortis, J. (Ed.): *Recent Advances in Biological Psychiatry*. New York, Plenum Press, 1963.

Brune, G.G. and Pscheidt, G.R.: Correlations between behavior and urinary excretion of indole amines and catecholamines in schizophrenic patients affected by drugs. *Fed. Proc.*, *20*:889-893, 1961.

Bumpus, F.M. and Page, I.H.: Serotonin and its methylated derivatives in human urine. *J. Biol. Chem.*, *212*:111-116, 1955.

Burckard, E., Medhaoui, M., Montigneaux, P., Pfitzenmeyer, J., Pfitzenmeyer, H., Schaetzel, J.C., Singer, L. and Geissmann, P.: Clinical, biological and electroencephalographic study of the action of tetrabenazine (RO 9569) in various chronic psychoses. *Ann. Medico. Psychol.*, *120*(1):115-119, 1962.

Buscaino, G.A., Spadetta, V. and Carella, A.: *In vitro* methylation of nicotinamide: a biochemical test for schizophrenia. In Lopez bor, J. (Ed.): Proceedings of the IVth World Congress of Psychiatry. Amsterdam, Excerpta Medica Foundation, 1966.

Buscaino, G.A. and Stefanachi, L.: Urinary excretion of 5-hydroxyindoleacetic acid in psychotic and normal subjects: excretion after parenteral administration of serotonin. *Arch. Neurol. Psychiat.*, *80*: 78-85, 1958.

Caffey, E.M., Diamond, L.S., Frank, T.V., Grasberger, J.C., Herman, L., Klett, C.J. and Rothstein, C.: Discontinuation or reduction of chemotherapy in chronic schizophrenics. *J. Chron. Dis.*, *17*:347-358, 1964.

Cagara, S. and Wozniak, M.: Clinical test of Frenolon. *Neurol. Neurochir. Psychiat. Pol.*, *16*:711-714, 1966.

Caldwell, A.E.: History of psychopharmacology. In Clark, W.G. and del Giudice, J. (Eds.): *Principles of Psychopharmacology*. New York, Academic Press, 1970a.

Caldwell, A.E.: Origins of Psychopharmacology from CPZ to LSD. Springfield, Thomas, 1970b.

Cancro, R. and Wilder, R.: A mechanism of sudden death in chlorpromazine therapy. *Amer. J. Psychiat.*, *127*(3):368-371, 1970.

Cannon, W.B.: *Bodily Changes in Pain, Hunger, Fear and Rage*. New York: Appleton, 1915.

Cantoni, G.L.: S-adenosylmethionine: a new intermediate formed enzymatically from l-methionine and adenosine-triphosphate. *J. Biol. Chem.*, *204*:403-416, 1953.

Cappelen, T. and Monrad, L.H.: Kliniske erfaringer med Truxal og Hibanil ved Kronisk schizofreni et double-forsk. *T. Norsk. Laegeforen, 81*:486-488, 1961.

Casey, J.F., Bennett, I.F., Lindley, C.J., Hollister, L.E., Gordon, M.H. and Springer, N.N.: Drug therapy in schizophrenia: a controlled study of the relative effectiveness of chlorpromazine, promazine, phenobarbital and placebo. *Arch. Gen. Psychiat.* 2:210-220, 1960a.

Casey, J.F., Hollister, L.E., Klett, C.J., Lasky, J.J. and Caffey, E.M.:

Combined drug therapy of chronic schizophrenics. Controlled evaluation of placebo, dextroamphetamine, imipramine, isocarboxazid and trifluoperazine added to maintenance doses of chlorpromazine. *Amer. J. Psychiat.*, *117*:997-1003, 1961.

Casey, J.F., Lasky, J.J., Klett, C.J. and Hollister, L.E.: Treatment of schizophrenic reactions with phenothiazine derivatives. *Amer. J. Psychiat.*, *117*:97-105, 1960b.

Cawley, R.H.: The present status of physical methods of treatment of schizophrenia. In Coppen, A. and Walk, A. (Eds.): *Recent Developments in Schizophrenia.* Ashford, Headley Brothers, 1967.

Cawley, L.M.: Evaluation of carphenazine in hospitalized schizophrenic women. *Dis. Nerv. Syst.*, *28*:126-130, 1967.

Chanoit, P.F., Collomb, H., Kato, M., Kristjansen, P., Kupka, K., Lebedev, B.A., Leme Lopes, J., Rossi, R., Shepherd, M. and Sivadon, P.: Epidemiology and sociological aspects. In Bobon, D.P., Janssen, P.A.J. and Bobon, Jean (Eds.): *The Neuroleptics.* Basel, S. Karger, 1970.

Charalampous, K.D. and Brown, S.: A clinical trial of α-methyl-para-tyrosine in mentally ill patients. *Psychopharmacologia, (Berlin) 11*: 422-429, 1967.

Charpentier, P., Gailliot, P., Jacob, R., Gaudechon, J. and Buisson, P.: Recherches sur les dimethylaminopropyl-N phenothiazines substituées. *C.R. Acad. Sci. (Paris)*, *235*:59-60, 1952.

Chien, Ching-Piao: Clinical trial of SK&F 14336 concentrate for chronic psychotics. *Curr. Ther. Res.*, *11*(1):15-21, 1969.

Chien, Ching-Piao, Mary Sah, Dubiel, Gail, C., and Leighmin L.: Double-blind study comparing the intramuscular usage of an acridan derivative, SK&F 14336, to chlorpromazine. *Curr. Ther. Res.*, *12*(1): 52-56, 1970.

Chouinard, G., Ban, T.A., Lehmann, H.E. and Ananth, J.V.: Fluspirilene in the treatment of chronic schizophrenic patients. *Curr. Ther. Res. 12*(9):604-608, 1970.

Chouinard, G., Lehmann, H.E. and Ban, T.A.: Pimozide in the treatment of chronic schizophrenic patients. *Curr. Ther. Res.*, *12*(9): 598-603, 1970.

Claghorn, J.L.: Psychopharmacologic characteristics of an indole compound—molindone. *Curr. Ther. Res.*, *11*(8):524-527, 1969.

Closs, K., Wad, N. and Ose, E.: The 'pink spot' in schizophrenia. *Nature*, *214*:483, 1967.

Cohen, G., Holland, B., Sha, J. and Goldenberg, M.: The stability of epinephrine and arterenol (norepinephrine) in plasma and serum:

a comparison of normal and schizophrenic subjects. *Acta Neurol. Psychiat., 80*:489, 1958.

Cohen, G., Holland, B., Sha, J. and Goldenberg, M.: Plasma concentrations of epinephrine and norepinephrine during intravenous infusions in man. *J. Clin. Invest., 38*:1935-1941, 1959.

Cole, J.O. and Davis, J.M.: Antipsychotic drugs. In Bellak, L. (Ed.): *The Schizophrenic Syndrome.* New York, Grune and Stratton, 1969.

Cole, J.O., Goldberg, S. and Davis, J.: Drugs in the treatment of psychosis: controlled studies. In Solomon, P. (Ed.): *Psychiatric Drugs.* New York, Grune and Stratton, 1966.

Courvoisier, S.: Pharmacodynamic basis for the use of chlorpromazine in psychiatry. *J. Clin. Exp. Psychopathol.* and *Quart. Rev. Psychiat. Neurol., 17*:25-37, 1956.

Courvoisier, S., Fournel, J., Ducrot, R., Kolsky, M. and Koetschet, P.: Propriétés pharmacodynamiques du chlorhydrate de chloro-3-(diméthyl-amino-3'-propyl)-10-phénothiazine (4560 RP). Etude expérimental d'un nouveau corps utilisé dans l'anesthésie potentialisée et dans l'hibernation artificielle. *Arch. Int. Pharmacodyn., 92*: 305-361, 1953.

Curry, S.H., Davis, J.M., Janowsky, D.S. and Marshall, J.H.L.: Factors affecting chlorpromazine plasma levels in psychiatric patients. *Arch. Gen. Psychiat., 22*(3):209-215, 1970a.

Curry, S.H., Marshall, J.H.L., Davis, J.M. and Janowsky, D.S.: Chlorpromazine plasma levels and effects. *Arch. Gen. Psychiat. 22*(4): 289-296, 1970b.

Dabrowski, K.: *Positive Disintegration.* Boston, Little, Brown, 1964.

Dabrowski, K.: *Personality Shaping Through Positive Disintegration.* Boston, Little, Brown, 1967.

Dehnel, L.L., Vestre, N.D. and Schiele, B.C.: A controlled comparison of clopenthixol and perphenazine in a chronic schizophrenic population. *Curr. Ther. Res., 10*(4):169-176, 1968.

deJong, H. (1931): In deJong, H.: *Experimental Catatonia.* Baltimore, Williams & Wilkins, 1945.

Delay, J. and Deniker, P.: 38 cas de psychoses traitées par la cure prolongée et continué de 4560 RP. *C.R. Congr. Alièn. Neurol.* (France), *50*:497-502, 1952.

deVerteuile, R., Lehmann, H.E., Ban, T.A. and Saxena, B.M.: Fluphenazine enanthate in the treatment of hospitalized chronic psychotic patients: a controlled study. *Int. J. Clin. Pharmacol. 4*(2):219-222, 1971.

DiMascio, A. and Shader, R.I.: Drug administration schedules. *Amer. J. Psychiat.*, *126*(6):796-801, 1969.

Dohan, F.C., Grasberger, J.C., Lowell, F.M., Johnston, H.T. and Arbegast, Ann W.: Relapsed schizophrenics: more rapid improvement on a milk- and cereal-free diet. *Brit. J. Psychiat.*, *115*:595-561, 1969.

Domino, E.F.: Pharmacological analysis of the pathobiology of schizophrenia. In Siva Sankar, D.V. (Ed.): *Schizophrenia: Current Concepts and Research.* Hicksville, P.J.D. Publications, 1969.

Dynes, J.B.: Diabetes in schizophrenia and diabetes in nonpsychotic medical patients. *Dis. Nerv. Syst.*, *30*:341-344, 1969.

Efron, D.H.: Biochemistry of psychoses. Exp. Med. Surg., Suppl. 124, 1965.

Ekdawi, M.Y.: Changes in ward behavior of severely disabled schizophrenic patients: a four years' study. *Brit. J. Psychiat.* *112*:265-267, 1966.

Ellerbrook, R.C. and Purdy, M.D.: Capacity of stressed humans under mega dosages of nicotinic acid to synthesize methylated compounds. *Dis. Nerv. Syst.*, *31*(3):196-197, 1970.

Engelhardt, D.M., Freedman, N., Glick, B.S., Hankoff, L.D., Mann, D. and Margolis, R.: Prevention of psychiatric hospitalization with use of psychopharmacological agents. *J.A.M.A.*, *173*:147-149, 1960.

Engelhardt, D.M., Freedman, N., Rosen, B., Mann, D. and Margolis, R.: Phenothiazines in prevention of psychiatric hospitalization. *Arch. Gen. Psychiat.*, *11*:162-169, 1964.

Engelhardt, D.M. and Margolis, R.A.: Hospitalization of schizophrenic patients: prediction and prevention. In Rothman, T. (Ed.): *Changing Patterns in Psychiatric Care.* New York, Crown Publishers, 1970.

Engelhardt, D.M., Rosen, B., Freedman, N., Mann, D. and Margolis, R.: Phenothiazines in prevention of psychiatric hospitalization: II. Duration of treatment exposure. *J.A.M.A.*, *186*:981-983, 1963.

Engelhardt, D.M., Rosen, B., Freedman, N. and Margolis, R.: Phenothiazines in prevention of psychiatric hospitalization. *Arch. Gen. Psychiat.*, *16*:98-101, 1967.

Erlenmeyer-Kimling, L., Nicol, Susan, Rainer, J.D. and Edwards Deming, W.: Changes in fertility rates of schizophrenic patients in New York State. *Amer. J. Psychiat.*, *125*(7):916-927, 1969.

Evangelakis, M.G.: De-institutionalization of patients. *Dis. Nerv. Syst.*, *22*:26-32, 1961.

Evensen, H.: Recherches faites après la sortie sur environ 800 cas de démence précoce. Presented at the Sixth Congr. of Scandinavian Psychiatrists, Copenhagen, 1936.

100   *Schizophrenia: A Psychopharmacological Approach*

Evensen, H. (1904): Dementia Praecox. In Ödegard, O.: Changes in the prognosis of functional psychoses since the days of Kraepelin. *Brit. J. Psychiat., 113*:813-822, 1967.

Fabing, H.D. and Hawkins, J.R.: Intravenous bufotenine injection in human beings. *Science, 123*:886-887, 1956.

Faurbye, A.: The role of amines in the etiology of schizophrenia. *Comp. Psychiat., 9*(2):155-177, 1968.

Faurbye, A. and Pind, K.: Investigation on the occurrence of the dopamine metabolite 3,4-dimethoxyphenylethylamine in the urine of schizophrenics. *Acta Psychiat. Scand., 40*:240-243, 1964.

Feldman, P.E.: Clinical evaluation of benzquinamide (P-2647) in the control of tension states and "hypersyndromes". *Psychosomatics, 3*: 148-151, 1962.

Feldstein, A.: On the relationship of adrenalin and its oxidation products to schizophrenia. *Amer. J. Psychiat., 116*:454-456, 1959.

Feldstein, A.: Biochemical aspects of schizophrenia and antipsychotic drugs. In DiMascio, A. and Shader, R. (Eds.): *Clinical Handbook of Psychopharmacology*. New York, Science House, 1970.

Feldstein, A., Hoagland, H. and Freeman, H.: Radioactive serotonin in relation to schizophrenia. *Arch. Gen. Psychiat., 5*:246-251, 1961.

Felger, H.L.: Depressed hospitalized psychiatric patients treated with chlorprothixene concentrate. *J. New Drugs, 5*:240-248, 1965.

Fieve, R.R., Blumenthal, Bernice, and Little, Barbara: The relationship of atypical lymphocytes, phenothiazines and schizophrenia. *Arch. Gen. Psychiat., 15*:529-534, 1966.

Fincle, L.P. and Johnson, C.C.: Psychiatric and behavioral effects of chlorprothixene concentrate suspension in chronic hospitalized schizophrenics. *Dis. Nerv. Syst., 26*:225-228, 1965.

Fink, M., Shaw, R., Gross, G.E. and Coleman, F.S.: Comparative study of chlorpromazine and insulin coma in therapy of psychosis. *J.A.M.A. 166*:1846-1850, 1958.

Fischer, E., Fernandez, T.A., Vazquez, A.J. and DiStefano, A.O.: A bufotenin-like substance in the urine of schizophrenics. *J. Nerv. Ment. Dis., 133*:441-444, 1961.

Foucault, M.: *Madness and Civilization*. (Translated by Richard Howard). New York, Random House, 1965.

Fouks, L., Périvier, E., Gilbert, A., Houssait, A. and Lerno, M.: Reflections of a chemotherapeutist on nosology. *Ann. Med. Psychol., 24*:503-508, 1966.

Freeman, H.: The therapeutic value of combinations of psychotropic drugs: a review. *Psychopharmacol. Bull., 4*:1-27, 1967.

Freeman, H., Oktem, N. and Oktem, M.R.: A double blind study of SKF 14336 vs trifluoperazine in schizophrenic patients. *Curr. Ther. Res.*, *10*(10):537-542, 1968.

Freyhan, F.A.: Course and outcome of schizophrenia. *Amer. J. Psychiat.*, *112*:161-169, 1955.

Friedhoff, A.: Dopamine and mescaline metabolism. Presented at the Ninth Annual Meeting of the ACNP, San Juan, 1970.

Friedhoff, A.J. and Hollister, L.E.: Comparison of the metabolism of 3,4-dimethoxyphenylethylamine and mescaline in humans. *Biochem. Pharmacol 15*:269-273, 1966.

Friedhoff, A.J. and Van Winkle, E.: Isolation and characterization of a compound from the urine of the schizophrenic. *Nature, 194*:897-898, 1962.

Gaddum, J.H. (1954): In: Smythies, J.R.: Introduction. In Himwich, H.E., Kety, S.S. and Smythies, J.R. (Eds.): *Amines and Schizophrenia*. London, Pergamon Press, 1967.

Galbrecht, C.R. and Klett, C.J.: Predicting response to phenothiazine: the right drug for the right patient. *J. Nerv. Ment. Dis., 147*:173-183, 1968.

Gallant, D.M. and Bishop, M.P.: Cinanserin (SQ 10,643): a preliminary evaluation in chronic schizophrenic patients. *Curr. Ther. Res., 10*(9):461-463, 1968.

Gallant, D.M. and Bishop, M.P.: AHR-1900: a butyrophenone derivative. *Curr. Ther. Res., 11*(12):793-795, 1969.

Gallant, D.M., Bishop, M.P. and Guerrero-Figueroa, R.: AL-449: a preliminary evaluation of a new butyrophenone derivative in chronic schizophrenic patients. *Curr. Ther. Res., 10*(5):244-246, 1968.

Gantt, W.H.: Normal and abnormal adaptations—homeostasis, schizokinesis and autokinesis. *Dis. Nerv. Syst., 18*:30-33, 1957.

Gantz, R.S. and Birkett, D.P.: Phenothiazine reduction as a cause of rehospitalization. *Arch. Gen. Psychiat., 12*:586-588, 1965.

Garattini, S. and Valzelli, L.: *Serotonin*. Amsterdam, Elsevier, 1965.

Gardos, G., Rapkin, R.M. and DiMascio, A.: Trifluoperazine and chlorpromazine in combination and individually. *Curr. Ther. Res., 10*(12):609-612, 1968.

Garry, J.W. and Leonard, T.J.: Haloperidol: a controlled trial in chronic schizophrenia. *J. Ment. Sci., 108*:105-107, 1962.

Gastaut, H.: Etat actuel des connaissances sur l'electroencephalographie du conditionnement. *Electroenceph. Clin. Neurophysiol.*, supp. 6, 1957.

Gershon, S., Hekimian, L.J., Floyd, A. Jr. and Hollister, L.E.: α-Methyl-p-tyrosine (AMT) in schizophrenia. *Psychopharmacologia (Berlin)*, *11*:189-194, 1967.

Goldberg, S.C., Klerman, G.L. and Cole, J.O.: Changes in schizophrenic psychopathology and ward behavior as a function of phenothiazine treatment. *Brit. J. Psychiat.*, *111*:120-133, 1965.

Goldberg, S.C.: Prediction of response to antipsychotic drugs. In: Efron, D.H. (Ed.): *Psychopharmacology*. A Review of Progress 1957-1967. PHSP No. 1836. Washington, U.S. Government Printing Office, 1968.

Goldberg, S.C., Mattsson, N., Cole, J.O. and Klerman, G.L.: Prediction of improvement in schizophrenia under four phenothiazines. *Arch. Gen. Psychiat.*, *16*:107-117, 1967.

Goldstein, M., Anagnoste, B., Lauber, E. and McKereghan, M.R.: Inhibition of dopamine-β-hydroxylase by disulfiram. *Life Sci.*, *3*: 763-767, 1964.

Good, W.W., Sterling, M. and Holtzman, W.H.: Termination of chlorpromazine with schizophrenic patients. *Amer. J. Psychiat. 115*: 443-448, 1958.

Gorham, D.R. and Pokorny, A.D.: Effects of a phenothiazine and/or group psychotherapy with schizophrenics. *Dis. Nerv. Syst.*, *25*: 77-86, 1964.

Gottschalk, L.A., Gleser, G.C., Cleghorn, J.M., Stone, W.N. and Winget, Carolyn N.: Prediction of changes in severity of the schizophrenic syndrome with discontinuation and administration of phenothiazines in chronic schizophrenic patients: language as a predictor and measure of change in schizophrenia. *Comp. Psychiat.*, *11*(2):123-140, 1970.

Green, D.E. and Forrest, Irene S.: In vivo metabolism of chlorpromazine. *Canad. Psychiat. Ass. J.*, *11*:299-302, 1966.

Green, D.E. and Richter, D.: Adrenalin and adrenochrome. *Biochem. J.*, *31*:596-616, 1937.

Greenblatt, M.: Foreword. In May, P.R.A. (Ed.): *Treatment of Schizophrenia*. New York, Science House, 1968.

Greenblatt, M., Solomon, M.H., Evans, A.S. and Brooks, G.W.: Drug and social therapy in chronic schizophrenia. Springfield, Thomas, 1965.

Greiner, A.C.: Schizophrenia and the pineal gland. *Canad. Psychiat. Ass. J.*, *15*:433-447, 1970.

Greiner, A.C. and Nicolson, G.A.: Schizophrenia—melanosis—cause or side effect. *Lancet*, *ii*:1165-1167, 1965.

Grinspoon, W. and Ewalt, J.R.: A study of long-term treatment of chronic schizophrenia. Presented at the IVth World Congress of Psychiatry, Madrid, 1966.

Grinspoon, L., Ewalt, J.R. and Shader, R.: Psychotherapy and pharmacotherapy in chronic schizophrenia. *Amer. J. Psychiat.*, *124*(12): 1645-1652, 1968.

Grof, S., Vojtechovsky, M., Vitek, M. and Prankova, S.: Clinical and experimental study of the central effects of adrenochrome. *J. Neuropsychiat.*, *5*:33-50, 1963.

Gross, M., Hitchman, I.L., Reeves, W.P., Lawrence, J. and Newell, P.C.: Discontinuation of treatment with ataractic drugs. *Amer. J. Psychiat.*, *116*:931-932, 1960.

Haase, H.J., Frank, T., Knaack, M., Lehnhardt, C. and Richter-Peill, H.: Klinische Prüfung eines neuen Langzeitneurolepticums (Fluspirilene) unter besonderer Berüksichtigung der neuroleptischen Schwelle, *Nervenarzt*, *39*:275, 1968.

Hagopian, V., Stratton, D.B. and Busiek, R.D.: Five cases of pigmentary retinopathy associated with thioridazine administration. *Amer. J. Psychiat.*, *123*(1):97-100, 1966.

Hakim, R.A.: Indigenous drugs in the treatment of mental diseases. Presented at the Sixth Gujurate and Saurashtra Provincial Medical Conference, Baroda, 1953.

Hall, P., Hartridge, G. and Leeuwen van, G.H.: Effect of catechol O-methyl transferase in schizophrenia. *Arch. Gen. Psychiat.*, *20*:573-575, 1969.

Hamon, J., Paraire, J. and Velluz, J.: Remarques sur l'action du 4560 RP sur l'agitat on maniaque. *Ann. Medicopsychol.* (*Paris*), *110*-(1):331-335, 1952.

Hanlon, T.E., Nussbaum, K., Wittig, B., Hanlon, D.D. and Kurland, A.A.: The comparative effectiveness of amitriptyline, perphenazine, and their combination in the treatment of chronic psychotic female patients. *J. New Drugs*, *4*:52-60, 1964.

Hare, E.H. and Willcox, D.R.C.: Do psychiatric inpatients take their pills? *Brit. J. Psychiat.*, *113*:1435-1439, 1967.

Harley-Mason, J. (1952): In Osmond, H. and Smythies, J.: *Schizophrenia: A New Approach. J. Ment. Sci.*, *98*:309-315, 1952.

Haydu, G.G., Dhrymiotis, A., Korenyi, O. and Goldschmidt, L.: Effects of methionine and hydroxychloroquine in schizophrenia. *Amer. J. Psychiat.*, *122*:560-564, 1965.

Heath, R.G., Nesselhof, W., Bishop, M.P. and Byers, L.W.: Behavioral and metabolic changes associated with administration of tetraethylthiuram disulfide. *Dis. Nerv. Syst.*, *26*:99-105, 1965.

Heath, R.G., Nesselhof, W. and Timmons, E.: D'l-methionine-d, l-sulphoximine effects in schizophrenic patients. *Arch. Gen. Psychiat.*, *14*:213-217, 1966.

Hekimian, L.J., Floyd, A. and Gershon, S.: Clinical trial of an acridane derivative (SKF#14,336) in male schizophrenics. *Curr. Ther. Res.* *9*(1):17-23, 1967.

Herkert, E.E. and Keup, W.: Excretion patterns of tryptamine, indole-acetic acid, and 5-hydroxyindoleacetic acid, and their correlation with mental changes in schizophrenic patients under medication with alpha methyldopa. *Psychopharmacologia* (*Berlin*), *15*:48-59, 1969.

Hess, S.M., Connamacher, R.H., Ozaki, M. and Udenfriend, S.: The effects of alpha-methyldopa and alpha-methyltyrosine on the metabolism of norepinephrine and serotonin *in vivo*. *J. Pharmacol. Exp. Ther.*, *134*:129-138, 1961.

Hobbs, C.E., Wanklin, J. and Ladd, K.B.: Changing patterns of mental hospital discharges and readmissions in the past two decades. *Canad. Med. Ass. J.*, *93*:17-20, 1965.

Hoehn-Saric, R. and Gross, M.: Auditory hallucinations in schizophrenia: early changes under drug treatment and drug withdrawal. *Amer. J. Psychiat.*, *124*(8):1132-1135, 1968.

Hoenig, J.: The prognosis of schizophrenia. In Coppen, A. and Walk, A. (Eds.): *Recent Developments in Schizophrenia*. Ashford, Headley Brothers, 1967.

Hoenig, J. and Hamilton, M.W.: The schizophrenic patient under new management. *Comp. Psychiat.*, *7*:81-91, 1966.

Hoffer, A.: Adrenochrome in blood plasma. *Amer. J. Psychiat*, *114*:752-753, 1958.

Hoffer, A.: Adrenaline metabolites in schizophrenia. *Dis. Nerv. Syst.*, *21*(2):79-86, 1960.

Hoffer, A.: The adrenochrome theory of schizophrenia: a review. *Dis. Nerv. Syst.*, *25*:173-178, 1964.

Hoffer, A.: Enzymology of hallucinogens. *Int. J. Neuropsychiat.*, *2*:43, 1965.

Hoffer, A.: Enzymology of hallucinogens. In Martin, G.J. and Kisch, B. (Eds.): *Enzymes in Mental Health*. Philadelphia, Lippincott, 1966.

Hoffer, A.: The adrenochrome theory of schizophrenia: a review. *Dis. Nerv. Syst.*, *25*:173-178, 1969.

Hoffer, A. and Kenyon, M.: Conversion of adrenalin to adrenolutin in human blood serum. *Arch. Neurol. Psychiat.*, *77*:437-438, 1957.

Hoffer, A. and Osmond, H.: Scurvy and schizophrenia. *Dis. Nerv. Syst.*, *24*(5):273-285, 1963.

Hoffer, A., Osmond, H. and Smythies, J.: Schizophrenia: a new approach. *J. Ment. Sci.*, *100*:29-54, 1954.

Hogarty, G.E. and Gross, M.: Preadmission symptom differences between first admitted schizophrenics in the predrug and postdrug era. *Comp. Psychiat.* 7(2):134-140, 1966.

Hollister, L.E.: Clinical use of psychotherapeutic drugs: current status. *Clin. Pharmacol. Ther.*, *10*(2):170-198, 1970a.

Hollister, L.E.: Choice of antipsychotic drugs. *Amer. J. Psychiat.*, *127*-(2):186-190, 1970b.

Hollister, L.E. and Friedhoff, A.J.: Effects of 3,4-dimethoxyphenylethylamine in man. *Nature*, *210*:1377-1378, 1966.

Hollister, L.E. and Hall, R.A.: Phenothiazine derivatives and morphologic changes in the liver. *Amer. J. Psychiat.*, *123*(2):211-212, 1966.

Hollister, L.E., Moore, F.F., Forrest, F. and Bennett, J.L.: Antipyridoxine effect of d-penicillamine in schizophrenic men. *Amer. J. Clin. Nutr.*, *19*:307-312, 1966.

Hollister, L.E., Overall, J.E., Bennett, J.L., Kimbell, I. and Shelton, J.: Specific therapeutic actions of acetophenazine, perphenazine and benzquinamide in newly admitted schizophrenic patients. *Clin. Pharmacol. Ther.*, *8*:249-255, 1967.

Hollister, L.E., Overall, J.E., Caffey, E., Bennett, J.L., Meyer, F., Kimbell, I. and Honigfeld, G.: Controlled comparison of haloperidol with thiopropazate in newly admitted schizophrenics. *J. Nerv. Ment. Dis.*, *135*:544-549, 1962.

Hollister, L.E., Overall, J.E., Meyer, F. and Shelton, J.: Perphenazine combined with amitriptyline in newly admitted schizophrenics. *Amer. J. Psychiat.*, *120*:591-592, 1963.

Holmboe, R. and Astrup, C.: A follow-up study of 255 patients with acute schizophrenia and schizophreniform psychoses. *Acta Psychiat. Scand.* suppl. 115, 1957.

Huber, G.: Grenzen der psychiatrischen Pharmakotherapie bei der Behandlung chronisch Schizophrener. In Kranz, H. and Heinrich, K. (Eds.): *Begleitwirkungen und Misserfolge der psychiatrischen Pharmakotherapie*. Stuttgart, Georg Thieme Verlag, 1964.

Huntsman, A.G.: Scientific research versus the theory of probabilities. *Science*, *110*:566, 1949.

Hsu, J.J., Nol, E., Martinez, Maria L., Lessien, B., Paragas, P.G., Puhac, Maria and Braun, R.A.: One year study of fluphenazine enanthate. *Dis. Nerv. Syst.*, *28*:807-811, 1967.

Israelstam, D.M., Johnson, A. and Winchell, H.S.: Methionine and schizophrenia. *J. Nucl. Med.*, *8*:325-326, 1967.

Israelstam, D.M., Sargent, T., Finley, N.N., Winchell, H.E., Fish, M.B., Motto, J., Pollycove, M. and Johnson, A.: Abnormal methionine metabolism in schizophrenic and depressive states: a preliminary report. *J. Psychiat. Res.*, 7:185-190, 1970.

Janssen, P.A.J.: The evolution of the butyrophenones, haloperidol and meperidol from meperidine-like 4-phenylpiperidines. *Int. Rev. Neurobiol.*, 8:221-263, 1965.

Janssen, P.A.J., Jageneau, A.H., Demoen, P.J., Van de Westeringh, C., de Canniere, J.H., Raeymaekers, A.H., Wouters, M.S., Sanczuk, S. and Hermans, B.K.: Compounds related to pethidine. III. Basic ketones derived from norpethidine. *J. Med. Pharm. Chem.*, 2:271-280, 1960.

Janssen, P.A.J., Niemegeers, C.J. and Schellekens, K.H.: Pimozide, a chemically novel, highly potent and orally long-acting neuroleptic drug. I. The comparative pharmacology of pimozide, haloperidol and chlorpromazine. *Arzneimittelforschung, 18*:261-279, 1968.

Janssen, P.A.J., Van de Westeringh, C., Jageneau, A.H., Demoen, P.J., Hermans, K.K., Van Daele, G.H., Schellekens, K.H., Van der Eycken, C.A. and Niemegeers, C.J.: Chemistry and pharmacology of CNS depressants related to 4-(4-hydroxy-4-phenyl-piperidino)-butyrophenone. I. Synthesis and screening data in mice. *J. Med. Pharm. Chem.*, 1:281-297, 1959.

Jarvik, M.E.: Drugs used in the treatment of psychiatric disorders. In Goodman, L.S. and Gilman, A. (Eds.): *The Pharmacological Basis of Therapeutics*. Toronto, Macmillan, 1965.

Jaspers, K.: *General Psychopathology* (Translated by Hoenig, J.) Manchester, Manchester University Press, 1962.

Kammerer, T., Singer, L., Geissmann, P., and Wetta, J.M.: Use of a new neuroleptic: tetrabenazine. Clinical biological and electroencephalographic results. *Ann. Med. Psychol. 120*(1):106-115, 1962.

Karkalas, Y.: Fluphenazine enanthate: a report of a clinical trial in psychotic patients. *Curr. Ther. Res., 10*(4):196-200, 1968.

Karon, B.P. and Vandenbos, G.R.: Experience, medication and the effectiveness of psychotherapy with schizophrenics. *Brit. J. Psychiat., 116*:427-428, 1970.

Karn, W.N., Mead, B.T. and Fishman, J.J.: Double-blind study of chlorprothixene (Taractan), a panpsychotropic agent. *J. New Drugs, 1*:72-79, 1961.

Kassay, G. and Pinter, Anna: A method to overcome therapeutic resistance to neuroleptic drugs in chronic schizophrenic patients. *Arzneimittelforschung 19*(3a):480-482, 1969.

Kelly, D.H.W. and Sargant, W.: Present treatment of schizophrenia—a controlled follow-up study. *Brit. Med. J. 1*:147-150, 1965.

Keskiner, A., Simeon, J., Fink, M. and Itil, T.M.: Long-acting phenothiazine (fluphenazine decanoate) treatment of psychosis. *Arch. Gen. Psychiat., 18*:477-481, 1968.

Kety, S.S.: Possible relation of central amines to behavior in schizophrenic patients. *Fed. Proc., 20*:894-896, 1961.

Kety, S.S.: Catecholamines in neuropsychiatric states. *Pharmacol. Rev., 18*:787-798, 1966.

Kety, S.S.: Current biochemical approaches to schizophrenia. *New Eng. J. Med., 276*:325-331, 1967.

Kety, S.S.: Biochemical etiologies: a review. In Cole, J.O. and Hollister, L.E. (Eds.): *Schizophrenia.* New York, Medcom, 1971.

Klaf, F.S. and Hamilton, J.G.: Schizophrenia—a hundred years ago and today. *J. Ment. Sci., 107*:819-828, 1961.

Klein, D.F. and Davis, J.M.: *Diagnosis and Drug Treatment of Psychiatric Disorders.* Baltimore, Williams & Wilkins, 1969.

Klett, C.J. and Moseley, E.C.: The right drug for the right patients. *J. Consult. Psychol., 29*:546-551, 1965.

Kline, N.S.: Use of *Rauwolfia serpentina Benth* in neuropsychiatric conditions. *Ann. New York Acad. Sci., 59*:107-132, 1954.

Kline, N.S.: Use of reserpine, the newer phenothiazines and iproniazid. *Res. Publ. Ass. Res. Nerv. Ment. Dis., 37*:218-244, 1959.

King, P.D.: Controlled study of group psychotherapy in schizophrenics receiving chlorpromazine. *Psychiat. Dig., 24*(1):21-23, 1963.

Korenyi, C. and Lowenstein, B.: Chlorpromazine-induced diabetes. *Dis. Nerv. Syst., 29*:827-828, 1968.

Korenyi, C.: The effect of benzophenone sunscreen lotion on chlorpromazine-treated patients. *Amer. J. Psychiat., 125*(7):971-974, 1969.

Kraepelin, E.: *Psychiatrie ein Lehrbuch für studierende und Arzte.* Leipzig, Barth, 1896 and 1910.

Krakoff, I.H.: Effect of methionine sulphoximine in man. *Clin. Pharm. Therap., 2*:559-604, 1961.

Kuehl, F.A., Hichens, M., Ormond, R.E., Preisinger, M.A.P., Gale, P.H., Cirillo, V.J. and Brink, N.G.: Para-O-methylation of dopamine in schizophrenic and normal individuals. *Nature, 203*:154-155, 1964.

Kuehl, F.A.: Para-O-methylation of dopamine in schizophrenics and normal individuals. In Himwich, H.E., Kety, S.S. and Smythies, J.R. (Eds.): *Amines in Schizophrenia.* Oxford, Pergamon Press, 1967.

Kurland, A.A.: Comparison of chlorpromazine and reserpine in treatment of schizophrenia. A study of four hundred cases. *Arch. Neurol. Psychiat.*, 75:510-513, 1956.

Kurland, A.A., Hanlon, T.E., Tatom, M.H., Oza, K.Y. and Simopoulos, A.M.: The comparative effectiveness of six phenothiazine compounds, phenobarbital and inert placebo in the treatment of acutely ill patients: global measures of severity of illness. *J. Nerv. Ment. Dis.*, 134:48-61, 1962.

Kurland, A.A. and Richardson, J.H.: A comparative study of two long acting phenothiazine preparations: fluphenazine-enanthate, and fluphenazine decanoate. *Psychopharmacologia (Berlin)*, 9:320-327, 1966.

Laborit, H.: L'hibernation artificielle. *Acta Chir. Belg.*, 50:710-715, 1951.

Laborit, H., Huguenard, P. and Alluame, R.: Un *nouveau* stabilisateur végétatif (le 4560 RP). *Presse Méd.*, 60:206-208, 1952.

LaBrosse, E.H., Mann, J.D. and Kety, S.S.: The physiological and psychological effects of intravenously administered epinephrine, and its metabolism in normal and schizophrenic men—III. Metabolism of 7-H3-epinephrine as determined in studies on blood and urine. *J. Psychiat. Res.*, 1:68-75, 1963.

Laestma, J.E. and Koenig, K.L.: Sudden death and phenothiazines. *Arch. Gen. Psychiat.*, 18:137-148, 1968.

Laing, R.D.: *The Politics of Experience*. London, Pelican Books, 1967.

Lampe, W.T.: A double-blind study of clomacran. *Curr. Ther. Res.*, 11(5):300-306, 1969.

Langfeldt, G.: The prognosis in schizophrenia and the factors influencing the course of the disease. *Acta Psychiat. Scand.*, suppl. 13, 1937.

Langsley, D.G., Enterline, J.D. and Hickerson, G.: A comparison of chlorpromazine and EST in treatment of acute schizophrenic and manic reactions. *Arch. Neurol. Psychiat.*, 81:384-391, 1959.

Lapierre, Y.D., Lapointe, L., Bordeleau, J.M. and Tetreault, L.: Phenothiazine treatment and electrocardiographic abnormalities. *Canad. Psychiat. Ass. J.*, 14:517-523, 1969.

Lasky, J.J., Klett, C.J., Caffey, E.M., Bennett, J.L., Rosenblum, M.D. and Hollister, L.E.: Drug treatment of schizophrenic patients: a comparative evaluation of chlorpromazine, chlorprothixene, fluphenazine, reserpine, thioridazine and triflupromazine. *Dis. Nerv. Syst.*, 23:698-706, 1962.

Leach, B.E. and Heath, R.G.: The *in vitro* oxidation of epinephrine in plasma. *Arch. Neurol. Psychiat.*, 76:444-450, 1956.

Lehmann, H.E.: Drug treatment of schizophrenia. In Kline, N.S. and

Lehmann, H.E. (Eds.): *Psychopharmacology*. Boston, Little, Brown, 1965.

Lehmann, H.E.: Pharmacotherapy of schizophrenia. In Hoch, P. and Zubin, J. (Eds.): *Psychopathology of Schizophrenia*. New York, Grune and Stratton, 1966.

Lehmann, H.E.: Problems in controlled clinical evaluation. In Efron, D.H. (Ed.): Psychopharmacology—a review of progress. P.H.S.P. No. 1836, Washington, U.S. Government Printing Office, 1968.

Lehmann, H.E.: The impact of the therapeutic revolution on nosology. In *Problems of Psychosis*. Excerpta Medica International Congress Series No. 194, 1969a.

Lehmann, H.E.: The impact of modern pharmacotherapy on the prognosis of psychiatric patients. *Transactions of the Association of Life Insurance Medical Directors of America*, *53*:31-47, 1969b.

Lehmann, H.E. and Ban, T.A. (Eds.): *The Butyrophenones in Psychiatry*. Montreal, Quebec Psychopharmacological Research Association, 1964a.

Lehmann, H.E. and Ban, T.A.: Notes from the log-book of a psychopharmacological research unit I. *Canad. Psychiat. Ass. J.*, *9*:28-32, 1964b.

Lehmann, H.E. and Ban, T.A.: Notes from the log-book of a psychopharmacological research unit II. *Canad. Psychiat. Ass. J.*, *9*:111-113, 1964c.

Lehmann, H.E. and Ban, T.A. (Eds.): *The Thioxanthenes*. Basel, S. Karger, 1969c.

Lehmann, H.E. and Ban, T.A.: Studies with thioxanthenes. In Lehmann, H.E. and Ban, T.A. (Eds.): *The Thioxanthenes*. Basel, S. Karger, 1969d.

Lehmann, H.E. and Ban, T.A.: Clinical use of other antipsychotic agents. In Clark, W.G. and del Giudice, J. (Eds.): *Principles of Psychopharmacology*. New York, Academic Press, 1970.

Lehmann, H.E., Ban, T.A., Matthews, V. and Garcia-Rill, T.: The effects of haloperidol on acute schizophrenic patients. A comparative study of haloperidol, chlorpromazine and chlorprothixene. In Lehmann, H.E. and Ban, T.A. (Eds.): *The Butyrophenones in Psychiatry*. Montreal, Quebec Psychopharmacological Research Association, 1964.

Lehmann, H.E. and Hanrahan, G.E.: Chlorpromazine, new inhibiting agent for psychomotor excitement and manic states. *Arch. Neurol. Psychiat.*, *71*:227-237, 1964.

Leonard, R.: Thioridazine in the plateaued patient. *Dis. Nerv. Syst.*, *29*:462-464, 1968.

Leonhard, K. (1936): Die Defectschizophrenen Krankheitsbilder, Leipzig. In Astrup, C.: *Schizophrenia: Conditional Reflex Studies.* Springfield, Thomas, 1962.

Letemendia, F.J.J. and Harris, A.D.: Chlorpromazine and the untreated chronic schizophrenic: a long term trial. *Brit. J. Psychiat., 113*:950-958, 1967.

Lingjaerde, O.: Tetrabenazine (Nitoman) in the treatment of psychoses. *Acta Psychiat. Scand., 39*:1-109, 1963.

Lucas, C.J., Sainsbury, P. and Collins, J.C.: A social and clinical study of delusions in schizophrenia. *J. Ment. Sci. 108*:747-758, 1962.

Madalena, J. C.: Um nôvo ataraxico de açào prolongada o R 6218 o contrôle dos seus effeitos extrapiramidais cum um nôvo agente antiparkinsoniano o R 4929. *Folha Med., 57*(6):943-958, 1968.

Mahler, H.R. and Cordes, E.H.: *Biological Chemistry.* New York, Harper and Row, 1966.

Malitz, S.: Pharmacological treatment. In Kolb, L.C., Kallmann, F.J. and Polatin, P. (Eds.): *Schizophrenia.* International Psychiatry Clinics, Vol. I, No. 4. Boston, Little, Brown, 1964.

Mandel, A. and Gross, M.: Agranulocytosis and phenothiazines. *Dis. Nerv. Syst., 29*:32-36, 1968.

Mandell, A.J. and Morgan, M.: Human brain enzyme makes indole hallucinogens. Presented at the 123rd Annual Meeting of the American Psychiatric Association, San Francisco, 1970.

Mann, J.C. and LaBrosse, F.H.: Urinary excretion of phenolic acid by normal and schizophrenic male patients. *Arch. Gen. Psychiat., 1*:547-551, 1959.

Markowe, M., Steinert, J. and Heyworth-Davis, F.: Insulin and chlorpromazine in schizophrenia: a ten year comparative survey. *Brit. J. Psychiat., 113*:1101-1106, 1967.

Marks, J.: Predrug behavior as a predictor of response to phenothiazines among schizophrenics. *J. Nerv. Ment. Dis., 137*:597-601, 1963.

May, P.R.A.: *Treatment of Schizophrenia: A Comparative Study of Five Treatment Methods.* New York, Science House, 1968.

May, P.R.A. and Tuma, A.H.: Treatment of schizophrenia. An experimental study of five treatment methods. *Brit. J. Psychiat., 111*:503-510, 1965.

McClelland, T.A. and Cowan, Gary: Use of antipsychotic and antidepressant drugs by chronically ill patients. *Amer. J. Psychiat. 126*-(12):1771-1773, 1970.

McDonald, R.K.: Problems in biologic research in schizophrenia. *J. Chron. Dis., 8*:366-371, 1958.

McDonald, R.K., Weise, V.K., Evans, F.T. and Patrick, R.C.: Studies on plasma ascorbic acid ceruloplasmin levels in schizophrenia. In Folch-Pi, J. (Ed.): *Chemical Pathology of the Nervous System.* Oxford, Pergamon Press, 1961.

McKenzie, M.E. and Roswell-Harris, D.: A controlled trial of prothi-pendyl (Tolnate) in mentally subnormal patients. *Brit. J. Psychiat.,* 112:95-100, 1966.

McKinney, W.J. Jr. and Kane, F.J. Jr.: Pancytopenia due to chlorpro-mazine. *Amer. J. Psychiat., 123*(7):879-880, 1967.

McNeill, D.L.M. and Madgwick, J.R.A.: A comparison of results in schizophrenics treated with (1) insulin (2) trifluoperazine (Stela-zine). *J. Ment. Sci.,* 107:297-299, 1961.

Medical Letter: Antipsychotic drugs and their major adverse effects. *Med. Letter Drugs Therapeutics, 12*(25):104, 1970.

Messier, M., Finnerty, R., Botvin, Constance S. and Grinspoon, L.: A follow-up study of intensively treated chronic schizophrenic pa-tients. *Amer. J. Psychiat., 125*(8):1123-1127, 1969.

Michaux, M.H., Kurland, A.A. and Agallianos, D.D.: Chlorpromazine-chlordiazepoxide and chlorpromazine-imipramine treatment of new-ly hospitalized, acutely ill psychiatric patients. *Curr. Ther. Res.,* 8:117-152, 1966.

Miller, J. and Daniel, G.R.: A trial of fluphenazine enanthate in chronic schizophrenia. *Brit. J. Psychiat.,* 113:1431-1432, 1967.

Miller, D.H., Clancy, J. and Cumming, E.: A comparison between uni-directional current non-convulsive electrical stimulation given with Reiter's Machine, standard alternating current electroshock (Cer-letti Method) and pentothal in chronic schizophrenia. *Amer. J. Psychiat.,* 109:617-620, 1953.

Morgan, D.W., Porzio, R.J. and Hedlund, J.L.: Schizophrenic symp-tom change with rehospitalization. *Arch. Gen. Psychiat.,* 19:227-231, 1968.

Morton, M.R.: A study of the withdrawal of chlorpromazine or trifluo-perazine in chronic schizophrenia. *Amer. J. Psychiat., 124*(11):1585-1588, 1968.

Mosher, L.R.: The center for studies of schizophrenia. *Schizophrenia Bull.,* 1:4-6, 1969.

Mueller, J.M., Schlittler, E. and Bein, H.J.: Reserpin, der sedative wirk-stoff aus Rauwolfia Serpentina Benth. *Experientia* 8:338-339, 1952.

Musacchio, J., Kopin, I.J. and Snyder, S.: Effects of disulfiram on tissue norepinephrine content and subcellular distribution dopamine, tyramine and their β-hydroxylated metabolites. *Life Sci.,* 3:769-775, 1964.

National Institute of Mental Health, Psychopharmacology Service Center Collaborative Study Group: Phenothiazine treatment in acute schizophrenia: Effectiveness. *Arch. Gen. Psychiat.*, *10*:246-261, 1964.

National Institute of Mental Health, Psychopharmacology Research Branch, Collaborative Study Group: Differences in clinical effects of three phenothiazines in "acute" schizophrenia. *Dis. Nerv. Syst.*, *28*:369-383, 1967.

Nemeth, J. and Petrovich, M.: Chlorpromazine and trifluoperazine treatment. *Dis. Nerv. Syst.*, *28*:812-814, 1967.

Nikolovski, O.T., Knowles, R.R. and Korol, B.: A clinical study of a new non-phenothiazine tranquilizer (SK&F 14336). *Curr. Ther. Res.*, *11*(4):178-181, 1969.

Nishimura, T. and Gjessing, L.R.: Failure to detect 3,4-dimethoxy-phenylethylamine and bufotenin in the urine from a case of periodic catatonia. *Nature*, *206*:963-964, 1965.

Noteboom, L.: Experimental catatonia by means of derivatives of mescaline and adrenaline. *Proc. Acad. Sci.*, *37*:562-574, 1934.

Nyirö, G.: The structural aspect of mental processes on the basis of reflex mechanisms. In Gegesi-Kiss, P. (Ed.): *Psychological Studies.* Budapest, Akademiai Kiado, 1958.

Ödegard, O.: Changes in the prognosis of functional psychoses since the days of Kraepelin. *Brit. J. Psychiat.*, *113*:813-822, 1967.

Ödegard, O.: The pattern of discharge and readmission in Norwegian mental hospitals, 1936-1963. *Amer. J. Psychiat.*, *125*(3):333-340, 1968.

Okasha, A. and Twefik, G.: Haloperidol: A controlled clinical trial in chronic disturbed psychotic patients. *Brit. J. Psychiat.*, *110*:56-60, 1964.

Oliveros, R.F., Amin, M., Ban, T.A and Lehmann, H.E.: A clinical trial of thiothixene in schizophrenics. *Curr. Ther. Res.*, *9*:504-507, 1967.

Oliveros, R.F., Ban T.A., Lehmann, H.E., Sterlin, C. and Saxena, B.M.: Thiothixene. Its range of therapeutic activity. *Int. J. Clin. Pharmacol.*, *3*(1):26-29, 1970.

Olson, G.W. and Peterson, D.B.: Sudden removal of tranquilizing drugs from chronic psychiatric patients. *J. Nerv. Ment. Dis.*, *131*: 252-255, 1960.

Oltman, Jane E. and Friedman, S.: Perphenazine-amitriptyline in the treatment of schizophrenia. *Amer. J. Psychiat.*, *123*(5):607-609, 1966.

Osmond, H. and Hoffer, A.: A comprehensive theory of schizophrenia.

Int. J. Neuropsychiat., 2(4):302-309, 1966.

Osmond, H. and Smythies, J.R.: Schizophrenia: a new approach. *J. Ment. Sci.*, 98:309-315, 1952.

Overall, J.E. and Gorham, D.R.: The Brief Psychiatric Rating Scale. *Psychol. Rep.*, 10:799-812, 1962.

Overall, J.E. and Hollister, L.E.: Psychiatric drug research sample size requirements for one versus two raters. *Arch. Gen. Psychiat.*, 16: 152-161, 1967.

Overall, J.E., Hollister, L.E., Bennett, J.L., Shelton, J. and Caffey, E.M.: Benzquinamide in newly admitted schizophrenics: a search for patients best treated with a specific drug. *Curr. Ther. Res.*, 5: 335-342, 1963a.

Overall, J.E., Hollister, L.E., Honigfeld, G., Kimbell, I.H., Meyer, F., Bennett, J.L. and Caffey, E.M.: Comparison of acetophenazine with perphenazine in schizophrenics: demonstration of differential effects based on computer-derived diagnostic models. *Clin. Pharmacol. Ther.*, 4:200-208, 1963b.

Pare, C.M., Sandler, M. and Stacey, R.S. (1958): In Garattini, S. and Valzelli, L.: *Serotonin.* Amsterdam, Elsevier, 1965.

Park, L.C., Baldessarini, R.J. and Kety, S.S.: Methionine effects on chronic schizophrenics. Patients treated with monoamine oxidase inhibitors. *Arch. Gen. Psychiat.*, 12:346-351, 1965.

Pavlov, I.P.: *Lectures on Conditioned Reflexes.* Translated by Gantt, W.H. New York, International Publishers, 1928.

Pearson, M.M.: Stecker's Fundamentals of Psychiatry. Montreal, Lippincott, 1963.

Pecknold, J.C., Ananth, J.V., Ban T.A. and Lehmann, H.E.: The use of methyldopa in schizophrenia: a review and comparative study. In press, 1971.

Perry, T.L., Hansen, S., and MacIntyre, L.: Failure to detect 3,4-dimethoxyphenylethylamine in the urine of schizophrenics. *Nature*, 202:519-520, 1964.

Perry, T.L., Hansen, S., MacDougall, L. and Schwartz, C.J.: Studies of amines in normal and schizophrenic subjects. In Himwich, H.E., Kety, S.S. and Smythies, J.R. (Eds.): *Amines and Schizophrenia.* Oxford, Pergamon Press, 1967.

Pind, K. and Faurbye, A.: The excretion of vanilmandelic acid in the urine of schizophrenics. *Scand. J. Clin. Lab. Invest.*, 13:288-290, 1961.

Platz, A.R., Klett, J. and Caffey, E.M., Jr.: Selective drug action related to chronic schizophrenic subtype. (A comparative study of carphenazine, chlorpromazine and trifluoperazine). *Dis. Nerv. Syst.*, *28*:601-605, 1967.

Pöldinger, W. and Schmidlin, P.: Index Psychopharmacorum, 1966. Verlag, Hans Huber Bern und Stuttgart, 1966.

Pollin, W., Cardon, P.V.J. and Kety, S.S.: Effect of amino acid feedings in schizophrenic patients treated with iproniazid. *Science, 133*: 104-105, 1961.

Prien, R.F. and Cole, J.O.: High dose chlorpromazine therapy in chronic schizophrenia. *Arch. Gen. Psychiat.*, *18*:482-495, 1968.

Prien, R.F., Cole, J.O. and Belkin, Naomi, F.: Relapse in chronic schizophrenics following abrupt withdrawal of tranquillizing medication. *Brit. J. Psychiat.*, *115*:679-686, 1968.

Pritchard, M.: Prognosis of schizophrenic before and after pharmacotherapy: I. Short term outcome. *Brit. J. Psychiat.*, *113*:1345-1352, 1967.

Pryce, I.G. and Edwards, H.: Persistent oral dyskinesia in female mental hospital patients. *Brit. J. Psychiat.*, *112*:983-987, 1966.

Pscheidt, G.R.: Excretion of catecholamines and exacerbation of symptoms in schizophrenic patients. *J. Psychiat. Res.*, *2*:163-168, 1964.

Pue, A.F., Hoare, R. and Adamson, J.D.: The 'Pink Spot' and schizophrenia. *Canad. Psychiat. Ass. J.*, *14*:397-401, 1969.

Radhakrishnan, K.C. and Chen, C.H.: Clinical trial of clomacran phosphate (SKF-14336) in chronic psychotic male patients. *Curr. Ther. Res.*, *12*(6):394-401, 1970.

Rahman, R.: A review of treatment of 176 schizophrenic patients in the mental hospital, Pabua. *Brit. J. Psychiat.*, *114*:775-777, 1968.

Ramsey, R.A., Lehmann, H.E., Ban, T.A., Saxena, B.M., and Bennett, Jean: A comparative study of molindone and trifluoperazine. *Curr. Ther. Res.*, *12*(7):438-440, 1970a.

Ramsey, R.A., Lehmann, H.E., Ban, T.A., Saxena, B.M. and Bennett, Jean: Clinical evaluation of a new psychotropic drug—molindone. *Int. J. Clin. Pharmacol.*, *3*(1):46-48, 1970b.

Randrup, A. and Munkvad, I.: On the measurement of adrenochrome in blood. *Amer. J. Psychiat.*, *117*:153, 1960.

Ravaris, C.L., Weaver, L.A. and Brooks, G.W.: Further studies with fluphenazine enanthate: II. Relapse rate in patients deprived of medication. *Amer. J. Psychiat.*, *124*(2):248-249, 1967.

Riddell, S.A.: The therapeutic efficacy of ECT. *Arch. Gen. Psychiat.*, *8*:546-556, 1963.

Rinaldi, F. and Himwich, H.E.: Drugs affecting psychotic behavior and the function of the mesodiencephalic activating system. *Dis. Nerv.*

Syst., *16*:133-141, 1955.

Rodnight, R.: Separation and characterization of urinary indoles resembling 5-hydroxytryptamine and tryptamine. *Biochem. J.*, *64*: 621, 1956.

Rosenberg, D.E., Isbell, H. and Miner, E.J.: Comparison of a placebo, N-dimethyltryptamine and 6-hydroxy-N-dimethyltryptamine in man. *Psychopharmacologia*, *4*:39-42, 1963.

Rossum Van, J.M.: Different types of sympathomimetic α-receptors. *J. Pharm. Pharmacol.*, *17*:202-216, 1965.

Roth, M.: Social implications of recent advances in psychopharmacology. *Brit. Med. Bull.*, *26*:197-202, 1970.

Rothstein, C., Zeltzerman, I. and White, H.R.: Discontinuation of ataractic drugs on a psychiatric continued treatment ward. *J. Nerv. Ment. Dis.*, *134*:555-560, 1962.

Roxburgh, P.A.: Treatment of persistent phenothiazine-induced oral dyskinesia. *Brit. J. Psychiat.*, *116*:277-280, 1970.

Ruck, F. and Schwarz, B.: Experiences regarding the effect of Frenolon in cases of schizophrenic psychoses. *Psychiat. Neurol. Med. Psychol.*, *17*:341-348, 1965.

Saarma, J.M.: Prognostic prediction of the insulin therapy of schizophrenia based on data on the higher nervous activity. Presented at the First Int. Congr. Social Psychiat. London, 1964.

Saarma, J.M.: Corticodynamics and treatment of schizophrenics. Tallin, Izdatelstvo "Valgys," 1970.

Saarma, J.M. and Vasar, H.: Nicotinic acid as an adjuvant in the treatment of chronic schizophrenic patients with special reference to changes in higher nervous activity. *Curr. Ther. Res.*, *12*(11):729-733, 1970.

Sai-Halasz, A., Brunecker, G. and Szara, S. (1958): In Faurbye, A.: The role of amines in the etiology of schizophrenia. *Comp. Psychiat.*, *9*(2):155-177, 1968.

Sainz, A.: Benzquinamide: a preliminary report. *Amer. J. Psychiat.*, *119*:777-778, 1963.

Sargant, W. and Slater, E.: An Introduction to Physical Methods of Treatment in Psychiatry. Livingstone, Edinburgh, 1963.

Scanlan, E.P. and May, A.E.: A controlled trial of Taractan in chronic schizophrenia. *Brit. J. Psychiat.*, *109*:418-421, 1963.

Scheff, T.J.: Schizophrenia as ideology. *Schizophrenia Bull.*, *2*:15-19, 1970.

Scheflen, A.E.: A psychotherapy of schizophrenia: direct analysis. Springfield, Thomas, 1961.

Schneider, C. (1942): The schizophrenen symptom verbände. Berlin. In: Astrup, C.: *Schizophrenia Conditional Reflex Studies.* Springfield, Thomas, 1962.

Schwarz, B.E., Sem-Jacobsen, C.W. and Petersen, M.C.: Effects of mescaline, LSD_{25}, and adrenochrome on depth electrograms in man. *Arch. Neurol. Psychiat.*, 75:579-587, 1956.

Scriabine, A., Weissman, A., Finger, K.F., Constantine, J.W. and Schneider, J.: Benzquinamide: a new anxiety drug. *J.A.M.A., 184:* 276-279, 1963.

Sen, N.P. and McGreer, P.L.: 4-methoxyphenylethylamine and 3,4-dimethoxyphenylethylamine in human urine. *Biochem. Biophys. Res. Commun., 14:*227-232, 1964.

Settel, E.: A clinical evaluation of benzquinamide with observations on the total activity potential. *Clin. Med., 70:*957-962, 1963.

Shawver, J.R., Gorham, D.R., Leskin, L.W., Good, W.W. and Kabnick, D.E.: Comparison of chlorpromazine and reserpine in maintenance drug therapy. *Dis. Nerv. Syst., 20:*452-457, 1959.

Shelton, J., Prusmack, J.J. and Hollister, L.E.: Molindone, a new type of antipsychotic drug. *J. Clin. Pharmacol., 8:*190-195, 1968.

Shelton, W.: SKF-10,812: a thioxanthene derivative. *Curr. Ther. Res.,* 7:415-416, 1965.

Shepherd, M.: A study of the major psychoses in an English county. London, Maudsley Monograph, 1957.

Sheppard, C. and Merlis, S.: Drug-induced extrapyramidal symptoms: their incidence and treatment. *Amer. J. Psychiat., 123*(7):886-889, 1967.

Shulgin, A.T., Sargent, T. and Naranjo, C.: A role of 3,4-dimethoxyphenylethylamine in schizophrenia. *Nature, 212:*1606-1607, 1966.

Siegler, M., Osmond, H. and Mann, H.: Laing's models of madness. *Brit. J. Psychiat., 115:*947-958, 1969.

Silverman, J.: When schizophrenia helps. *Psychology Today 4*(4):62-70, 1970.

Simon, W., Wirt, A.L., Wirt, R.D. and Halloran, A.V.: Long-term followup study of schizophrenic patients. *Arch. Gen. Psychiat., 12:*510-515, 1965.

Simon, W., Wirt, R.D., Wirt, A.L., Halloran, A.V., Hinckley, R.G., Lund, J.B. and Hopkins, G.W.: A controlled study of the short term differential treatment of schizophrenia. *Amer. J. Psychiat., 114:*1077-1086, 1958.

Simpson, G.M., Amin, M., Kunz, Esther, and McCafferty, F. Virginia: Studies on a second long-acting fluphenazine. *Amer. J. Psychiat., 121:*784-787, 1965.

Simpson, G.M., Angus, J.W.S. and Edwards, J.G.: A controlled study of haloperidol in chronic schizophrenia. *Curr. Ther. Res.*, *9*:407-412, 1967.

Simpson, G.M., Angus, J.W.S. and Edwards, J.G.: A preliminary study of C1-601 in chronic schizophrenia. *Curr. Ther. Res.*, *9*(9):486-491, 1967.

Simpson, G.M. and Angus, J.W.S.: A preliminary study of oxypendyl in chronic schizophrenia. *Curr. Ther. Res.*, *9*(4):225-228, 1967a.

Simpson, G.M. and Angus, J.W.S.: A preliminary study of prothipendyl in chronic schizophrenia. *Curr. Ther. Res.*, *9*(5):265-268, 1967b.

Simpson, G.M. and Krakov, L.: A preliminary study of molindone (EN-1733A) in chronic schizophrenia. *Curr. Ther. Res.*, *10*(1): 41-46, 1968.

Skarbek, A. and Hill, G.B.: An extended trial of oxypertine in five selected cases on chronic schizophrenia. *Brit. J. Psychiat.*, *113*:1107-1112, 1967.

Skarbek, A. and Jacobsen, M.: Oxypertine, a review of clinical experience. *Brit. J. Psychiat.*, *111*:1173-1179, 1965.

Smith, K., Surphlis, W.R.P., Gynther, M.D. and Shimkunas, A.M.: ECT-chlorpromazine and chlorpromazine compared in the treatment of schizophrenia. *J. Nerv. Ment. Dis.*, *144*:284-290, 1967.

Smith, K., Thompson, G.F. and Koster, H.: Sweat in schizophrenic patients: identification of the odorous substance. *Science*, *166*(3903): 398-399, 1969.

Smythies, J.R. (1960): In Garattini, S. and Valzelli, L. (Eds.): *Serotonin*. Amsterdam, Elsevier, 1965.

Smythies, J.R.: Recent advances in the biochemistry of schizophrenia. In Coppen, A. and Walk, A. (Eds.): *Recent Developments in Schizophrenia*. Ashford, Headley Brothers, 1967a.

Smythies, J.R.: Introduction. In: Himwich, H.E., Kety, S.S. and Smythies, J.R. (Eds.): *Amines in Schizophrenia*. Oxford, Pergamon Press, 1967b.

Smythies, J.R., and Sykes, E.A.: Structure-activity relationship of mescaline. In Himwich, H.E., Kety, S.S. and Smythies, J.R. (Eds.): *Amines and Schizophrenia*. Oxford, Pergamon Press, 1967.

Snezhnevski, A.V.: Psychopharmacology and psychiatry. *Int. J. Psychiat.*, *1*:219-228, 1965.

Spaide, J., Neveln, L., Tolentino, J. and Himwich, H.E.: Methionine and tryptophan loading in schizophrenic patients receiving a MAO Inhibitor: correlation of behavioral and biochemical changes. *Biol. Psychiat.*, *1*:227-235, 1969.

Sprince, H.: Indole metabolism in mental illness. *Clin. Chem.*, 7:203-230, 1961.

Sprince, H., Parker, C.M., Jameson, D. and Alexander, F.: Urinary indoles in schizophrenic and psychoneurotic patients after administration of tranylcypromine (Parnate) and methionine or tryptophan. *J. Nerv. Ment. Dis.*, 137:246-251, 1963.

Staehelin, J.E. and Kielholz, P.: Largactil, ein neues vegetatives Dämpfungsmittel bei psychischen Störungen. *Schweiz. Med. Wschr.*, 83: 581-586, 1953.

Stam, F.C., Heslinga, F.J.M., and Tilburg, van, W.: Schizophrenia and the pink spot. *Psychiat. Neurol. Neurochir.*, 72:513-524, 1969.

Steinberg, H.R., Green, R., and Durell, J.: Depression occurring during the course of recovery from schizophrenic symptoms. *J. Amer. Psychiat.*, 124(5):699-702, 1967.

Sterkmans, P., Brugmans, J. and Gevers, F.: The clinical efficacy of pimozide in chronic psychotic patients. *Clin. Trials J. (London)*, 5(4):1107, 1968.

Sterkmans, P., Brugmans, J. and Gevers, F.: Clinical evaluation of fluspirilene—oR 4929. *Folha Med.*, 57(6):943, 1969.

Sterlin, C., Ban, T.A., Lehmann, H.E. and Saxena, B.M.: The place of thiothixene in the treatment of schizophrenic patients. *Canad. Psychiat. Ass. J.*, 15:3-14, 1970.

Sterlin, C., Oliveros, R.F. and Ban, T.A.: Predictors of therapeutic responsivity to thiothixene in schizophrenics. *Int. J. Clin. Ther. Toxicol.*, 5:394-396, 1968.

Stern, E.S.: A statistical study of departures from a mental hospital. *Brit. J. Psychiat.*, 116:57-64, 1970.

Stewart, A.R. and Lavallee, B.: Fluphenazine enanthate for the difficult psychotic patient. *Dis. Nerv. Syst.*, 30:98-102, 1969.

St. Jean, A., Ban, T.A. and Noe, W.: Psychopharmacological studies with Neoserp and Aldomet. *Int. J. Neuropsychiat.*, 1(5):491-503, 1965.

St. Jean, A., Sterlin, C., Noe, W. and Ban, T.A.: Clinical studies with propericiazine (RP 8909). *Dis. Nerv. Syst.*, 28:526-531, 1967.

St. Laurent, J., Cahn, C.H. and Ban, T.A.: Treatment of psychiatric patients with a phenothiazine derivative (prochlorperazine) with special reference to after-care. *Amer. J. Psychiat.*, 118:938-940, 1962.

Stone, A.A., Hopkins, R., Mahnke, M.W., Shapiro, D.W. and Silverglate, H.A.: Simple schizophrenia syndrome or shibboleth. *Amer. J. Psychiat.*, 125(3):305-312, 1968.

Studnitz, W. and Nyman, G.E.: Excretion of 3,4-dimethoxyphenyl-ethylamine in schizophrenia. *Acta Psychiat. Scand., 41*:117-121, 1965.

Sugerman, A.A.: A pilot study of AL-449 in chronic schizophrenic patients. *Curr. Ther. Res., 10*(10):533-536, 1968.

Sugerman, A.A. and Herrmann, Jane: A pilot study of Dominal in chronic schizophrenics. *Curr. Ther. Res., 8*:487-489, 1966.

Sugerman, A.A. and Herrmann, Jane: Molindone: an indole derivative with antipsychotic activity. *Clin. Pharmacol. Therap. 8*:261-265, 1967.

Sugerman, A.A., Herrmann, Jane and O'Hara, Mary: A pilot study of AHR-1900 in chronic schizophrenic patients. *Curr. Ther. Res. 14* (4):234-236, 1970.

Sugerman, A.A., Lichtigfeld, F.J. and Herrmann, Jane: A pilot study of clopenthixol in chronic schizophrenics. *Curr. Ther. Res., 8*:220-224, 1966.

Sugerman, A.A., Williams, B.H. and Adlerstein, A.M.: Haloperidol in the psychiatric disorders of old age. *Amer. J. Psychiat., 120*:1190-1192, 1964.

Sulkowitch, H. and Altschule, M.D.: Urinary epinephrines in patients with mental and emotional disorders: apparent occurrence of adren-olutin-like substances in the urines of psychotic and depressed patients. *Arch. Gen. Psychiat., 1*:108-115, 1959.

Swanson, D.W., Smith, J.A. and Perez, H.: A fixed combination of chlorpromazine and trifluoperazine in psychotic patients. *Dis. Nerv. Syst., 28*:756, 1967.

Szara, S.: Dimethyltryptamine: Its metabolism in man: The relation of its psychotic effect to the serotonin metabolism. *Experientia, 12*: 441-442, 1956.

Szara, S.: Hallucinogenic effects and metabolism of tryptamine deriva-tives in man. *Fed. Proc., 20*:885-888, 1961.

Szara, S.: Hallucinogenic amines and schizophrenia. In Himwich, H.E., Kety, S.S. and Smythies, J.R. (Eds.): *Amines and Schizophrenia.* Oxford, Pergamon Press, 1967.

Szara, S., Axelrod, J. and Perlin, S.: Is adrenochrome present in the blood? *Amer. J. Psychiat., 115*:162, 1958.

Szasz, T.S.: *The Myth of Mental Illness.* New York, Harper Brothers, 1961.

Takesada, M., Kakimoto, Y., Sano, I. and Kaneko, Z.: 3,4-dimethoxy-phenylethylamine and other amines in the urine of schizophrenic patients. *Nature, 199*:203-204, 1963.

Tanimukai, H., Ginther, R., Spaide, J., Bueno, J. and Himwich, H.E.: Psychotomimetic indole compound in urine of schizophrenic and mentally defective patients. *Nature, 216*:490-491, 1967.

Tanimukai, H., Ginther, R., Spaide, J., Bueno, J.R. and Himwich, H.E.: Detection of psychotomimetic N, N-dimethylated indoleamines in the urine of four schizophrenic patients. *Brit. J. Psychiat., 117*: 421-430, 1970.

Tarasov, G.K.: Aminazine, review of the literature on the psychiatric use of a phenothiazine derivative. *Zh. Nevropat. Psikhiat. Korsakov, 55*:296-310, 1955.

Taubmann, G. and Jantz, H.: Untersuchung über dem Adrenochrom. Zugeschriebenen Psychotoxischen Wirkungen. *Nervenartz, 28*:485-488, 1957.

Tedeschi, D.H., Tedeschi, R.E. and Fellows, E.J.: Interaction of neuroleptics with serotonin in the central nervous system. *Rev. Canad. Biol., 20*:209-214, 1961.

Thonnard-Neumann, E.: Phenothiazines and diabetes in hospitalized women. *Amer. J. Psychiat., 124*(7):978-982, 1968.

Traugott, N.N., Bagrov, Y.Y., Balonov, L.Y., Deglin, V.L., Kaufman, D.A. and Lichko, A.F.: *Outlines of Psychopharmacology.* Leningrad, Nauka, 1968.

Turunen, S. and Salminen, J.: Neuroleptic treatment and mortality. *Dis. Nerv. Syst., 29*:474-477, 1968.

Tuteur, W., Stiller, R. and Glotzer, J.: Chlorpromazine: five years later. In Wortis, J. (Ed.): *Recent Advances in Biological Psychiatry.* New York, Grune and Stratton, 1961.

Usdin, E. and Efron, D.M.: Psychotropic drugs and related compounds. PHSP No. 1589, Washington, U.S. Government Printing Office, 1967.

Usdin, E. and Efron, D.M.: Psychotropic drugs and related compounds. PHSP No. 1589, Washington, U.S. Government Printing Office, 1969. (Supplement).

Varga, E.: *Changes in the Symptomatology of Psychotic Patterns.* Budapest, Akademiai Kiado, 1966.

Vartanian, F.E.: The change produced by treatment in the terminal stages of schizophrenia. *Zh. Nevropat. Psychiat. 66*:1571-1574, 1966.

Villeneuve, C., Ananth, J.V., Ban, T.A. and Lehmann, H.E.: CI-601, a butyrophenone derivative, in the treatment of chronically withdrawn schizophrenic patient. *Curr. Ther. Res., 12*(4):223-229, 1970.

Wagner, A.F., Cirillo, V.J., Meisinger, M.A.P., Ormond, R.E., Kuehl, F.A. and Brink, N.G.: A further study of catecholamine O-methylation in schizophrenia. *Nature, 211*:604-605, 1966.

Walker, R. and McCourt, J.: Employment experience among 200 schizophrenic patients in hospital and after discharge. *Amer. J. Psychiat.*, *122*:316-319, 1965.

Warnes, H., Canfield, Joyce and Ban, T.A.: An uncontrolled study with thiothixene. In Lehmann, H.E. and Ban, T.A. (Eds.): *The Thioxanthenes*. Basel, S. Karger, 1969.

Warnes, H., Lee, H., and Ban, T.A.: The comparative effectiveness of butyrophenones in chronic psychotic patients. In Lehmann, H.E. and Ban, T.A. (Eds.): *The Butyrophenones in Psychiatry*. Montreal, Quebec Psychopharmacological Research Association, 1964.

Warnes, H., Lehmann, H.E., Ban, T.A. and Lee, H.: Butaperazine and haloperidol: a comparative trial of two antipsychotic drugs. *Laval Med.*, *37*:143-145, 1966.

Watt, J.A.G., Aschcroft, G.W., Daly, R.J. and Smythies, J.R.: Urine volume and pink spots in schizophrenia and health. *Nature, 221*: 971-972, 1969.

Webb, R.R.: "Largactil" in psychiatry. *Med. J. Aust.*, *1*:759-761, 1955.

Weiner, D.N. and Feinberg, P.A.: Effects of withdrawal of tranquilizers from chronic psychiatric outpatient drug-users. Unpublished observations. In: Caffey, E.M., Diamond, L.S. and Frank, T.V.: Discontinuation or reduction of chemotherapy in chronic schizophrenics. *J. Chronic Dis.*, *17*:347-358, 1964.

Whittier, J.R., Korenyi, C., Haydu, G.G. and Goldschmidt, L.: Effects of long-acting injectable Prolixin in 23 psychotic patients. *Dis. Nerv. Syst.*, *28*:459-461, 1967.

Wiener, A.S.: Blood groups and disease. A critical review. *Lancet, 1*: 813-816, 1962.

Willis, J.H. and Bannister, D.: The diagnosis and treatment of schizophrenia. A questionnaire study of psychiatric opinion. *Brit. J. Psychiat.*, *111*:1165-1172, 1965.

Wing, J.K.: Social treatment, rehabilitation and management. In: Coppen, A. and Walk, A. (Eds.): *Recent Developments in Schizophrenia*. Ashford, Headley Brothers, 1967.

Wolpert, A., Sheppard, C. and Merlis, S.: An early clinical evaluation of clopenthixol in treatment resistant female schizophrenic patients. *Amer. J. Psychiat.*, *124*(5):702-705, 1967.

Woolley, D.W.: *The Biochemical Basis of Psychoses*. New York, Wiley, 1962.

Woolley, D.W. and Shaw, E.: A biochemical and pharmacological suggestion about certain mental disorders. *Science, 119*:587-588, 1954.

Wright, R.L.D. and Kyne, W.P.: A clinical and experimental comparison of four antischizophrenic drugs. *Psychopharmacologia 1*: 437-449, 1960.

Zelman, S. and Guillan, R.: Heat stroke in phenothiazine-treated patients: a report of three fatalities. *Amer. J. Psychiat.*, *126*(12):1787-1790, 1970.

AUTHOR INDEX

Achté, K.A., 30, 34, 51, 57
Ackner, B., 46
Adamson, J.D., 84
Adelson, D., 18, 19
Adlerstein, A.M., 20
Affleck, J.W., 81
Agallianos, D.D., 49
Albert, J.M., 69
Alexander, F., 87
Allen, J.L., 40
Alluaume, R., 4
Altschule, M.D., 83
Amin, M., 41
Ananth, J.V., 40, 75, 80, 87
Angus, J.W.S., 8, 20
Arnold, O.H., 78
Arthurs, D., 20
Ashcroft, G.W., 12
Astrachan, B.M., 57
Astrup, C., 51
Auch, W., 35
Axelrod, J., 79, 80, 83, 84, 87
Ayd, F.J., Jr., 5
Azima, H., 20

Baker, A.A., 47
Baldessarini, R.J., 87
Bankier, R.G., 48
Bannister, D., 16
Barker, P.A., 12
Bartolucci, G., 7
Battegay, R., 34, 57
Bein, H.J., 10
Benda, P., 77
Bergen, B., 48
Bergen, J.R., 85
Bergsman, A., 82
Berlet, H.H., 80, 87
Bertolotti, P., 12
Birkett, D.P., 37

Bishop, M.P., 8, 13, 23, 59, 78
Blackburn, H.L., 40
Bleuler, E.P., 57, 62
Bloom, J.B., 59
Blumenthal, Bernice, 59
Bobon, D.P., 14
Bohacek, N., 57
Bookhammer, R.S., 45
Borowski, T., 43
Bourdillon, R.E., 85
Bowers, M.B., Jr., 57
Brill, C., 80
Brill, H., vii, 31, 32, 33, 34, 35, 37, 38
Brodsky, L., 78
Brooks, G.W., 48
Brophy, J.J., 48
Brown, S., 81
Brugmans, J., 14
Brune, G.G., 79, 87
Brunecker, G., 78
Bumpus, F.M., 80
Burckard, E., 12
Buscaino, G.A., 77, 86, 88
Busiek, R.D., 59

Caffey, E.M., 25, 40
Cagara, S., 5
Cahn, C.H., 37
Caldwell, A.E., 3
Cancro, R., 42
Canfield, Joyce, 7
Cannon, W.B., 82
Cantoni, G.L., 87
Cappelen, T., 20
Cardon, P.V.J., 87, 88
Carella, A., 86, 88
Casey, J.F., 18, 19, 22, 23, 49
Cawley, R.H., vii, 16, 25, 26
Chanoit, P.F., 28, 43
Charalampous, K.D., 81

Gross, M., 37, 50, 55, 59
Guerrero-Figueroa, R., 13
Guillan, R., 60

Haase, H.J., 14
Hagopian, V., 59
Hakim, R.A., 10
Hall, P., 59, 88
Hamilton, J.G., 51, 53
Hamilton, M.W., 30, 37
Hamon, J., 3
Hanlon, T.E., 49
Hanrahan, G.E., 3
Hansen, S., 84
Hare, E.H., 49
Harley-Mason, J., 82, 85
Harris, A.D., 46
Hawkins, J.R., 78
Haydu, G.G., 88
Heath, R.G., 81, 83, 86
Hedlund, J.L., 50
Hekimian, L.J., 8
Herkert, E.E., 78
Herrmann, Jane, 7, 8, 13, 14
Heslinga, F.J.M., 85
Heyworth-Davis, F., 47
Hickerson, G., 47
Hill, G.B., 14
Himwich, H.E., 69, 79, 80, 87
Hoagland, H., 80
Hoare, R., 84
Hobbs, C.E., 34, 35
Hoehn-Saric, R., 55
Hoenig, J., 29, 30, 37
Hoffer, A., 82, 83, 84, 85
Hofmann, G., 78
Hogarty, G.E., 50
Hölderlin, 61
Hollister, L.E., 4, 14, 23, 26, 49, 59, 60, 66, 81, 85
Holmboe, R., 51
Holtzman, W.H., 40
Hsu, J.J., 48
Huber, G., 50
Huguenard, P., 4
Huntsman, A.G., 67

Isbell, H., 78
Israelstam, D.M., 86, 87

Jacobsen, C.W., 14, 83
Janssen, P.A.J., 12, 14
Jantz, H., 83
Jarvik, M.E., 4
Jaspers, K., 59, 61
Johnson, A., 86
Johnson, C.C., 20

Kammerer, T., 12
Kane, F.J., Jr., 59
Karkalas, Y., 48
Karn, W.N., 20
Karon, B.P., 46
Kassay, G., 76
Kelly, D.H.W., vii, 34, 47, 49, 50
Kenyon, M., 82, 83, 84
Keskiner, A., 48
Kety, S.S., 69, 82, 83, 85, 87, 88
Keup, W., 78
Kielholz, P., 3
King, P.D., 43
Klaf, F.S., 51, 53
Klein, D.F., vii, 5, 11, 18, 20, 21, 23
Klerman, G.L., 57, 58
Klett, C.J., 25, 26
Kline, N.S., 10
Knowles, R.R., 8
Koenig, K.L., 42
Kopin, I.J., 81
Korenyi, C., 60
Korol, B., 8
Koster, H., 87
Kraepelin, E., 28, 29, 30, 31, 51, 53, 62
Krakoff, I.H., 86
Krakov, L., 14
Kuehl, F.A., 85
Kurland, A.A., 11, 22, 23, 48, 49
Kyne, W.P., 11

Laborit, H., 4
LaBrosse, E.H., 82, 83
Ladd, K.B., 34, 35
Laestma, J.E., 42
Laing, R.D., 63
Langfeldt, G., 29, 30
Langsley, D.G., 47
Lampe, W.T., 8
Lapierre, Y.D., 59
Lasky, J.J., 23
Lavallee, B., 49

SUBJECT INDEX